T0227184

Psychological Issues in the ICU

Editor

DEBORAH W. CHAPA

CRITICAL CARE NURSING CLINICS OF NORTH AMERICA

www.ccnursing.theclinics.com

Consulting Editor
JAN FOSTER

December 2019 • Volume 31 • Number 4

ELSEVIER

1600 John F. Kennedy Boulevard • Suite 1800 • Philadelphia, Pennsylvania, 19103-2899

http://www.theclinics.com

CRITICAL CARE NURSING CLINICS OF NORTH AMERICA Volume 31, Number 4
December 2019 ISSN 0899-5885, ISBN-13: 978-0-323-68231-2

Editor: Kerry Holland
Developmental Editor: Laura Fisher

© **2019 Elsevier Inc. All rights reserved.**

This periodical and the individual contributions contained in it are protected under copyright by Elsevier, and the following terms and conditions apply to their use:

Photocopying

Single photocopies of single articles may be made for personal use as allowed by national copyright laws. Permission of the Publisher and payment of a fee is required for all other photocopying, including multiple or systematic copying, copying for advertising or promotional purposes, resale, and all forms of document delivery. Special rates are available for educational institutions that wish to make photocopies for non-profit educational classroom use. For information on how to seek permission visit www.elsevier.com/permissions or call: (+44) 1865 843830 (UK)/(+1) 215 239 3804 (USA).

Derivative Works

Subscribers may reproduce tables of contents or prepare lists of articles including abstracts for internal circulation within their institutions. Permission of the Publisher is required for resale or distribution outside the institution. Permission of the Publisher is required for all other derivative works, including compilations and translations (please consult www.elsevier.com/permissions).

Electronic Storage or Usage

Permission of the Publisher is required to store or use electronically any material contained in this periodical, including any article or part of an article (please consult www.elsevier.com/permissions). Except as outlined above, no part of this publication may be reproduced, stored in a retrieval system or transmitted in any form or by any means, electronic, mechanical, photocopying, recording or otherwise, without prior written permission of the Publisher.

Notice

No responsibility is assumed by the Publisher for any injury and/or damage to persons or property as a matter of products liability, negligence or otherwise, or from any use or operation of any methods, products, instructions or ideas contained in the material herein. Because of rapid advances in the medical sciences, in particular, independent verification of diagnoses and drug dosages should be made.

Although all advertising material is expected to conform to ethical (medical) standards, inclusion in this publication does not constitute a guarantee or endorsement of the quality or value of such product or of the claims made of it by its manufacturer.

Critical Care Nursing Clinics of North America (ISSN 0899-5885) is published quarterly by Elsevier Inc., 360 Park Avenue South, New York, NY 10010-1710. Months of issue are March, June, September, and December. Business and Editorial Offices: 1600 John F. Kennedy Blvd., Suite 1800, Philadelphia, PA 19103-2899. Periodicals postage paid at New York, NY and additional mailing offices. Subscription prices are $160.00 per year for US individuals, $406.00 per year for US institutions, $100.00 per year for US students and residents, $206.00 per year for Canadian individuals, $510.00 per year for Canadian institutions, $230.00 per year for international individuals, $510.00 per year for international institutions and $115.00 per year for Canadian and international students/residents. To receive student/resident rate, orders must be accompanied by name of affiliated institution, data of term, and the *signature* of program/residency coordinator on institution letterhead. Orders will be billed at individual rate until proof of status is received. Foreign air speed delivery is included in all *Clinics* subscription prices. All prices are subject to change without notice. **POSTMASTER:** Send address changes to *Critical Care Nursing Clinics of North America*, Elsevier Health Sciences Division, Subscription Customer Service, 3251 Riverport Lane, Maryland Heights, MO 63043. **Customer Service: 1-800-654-2452 (US and Canada); 314-447-8871 (outside US and Canada). Fax: 314-447-8029. E-mail:** JournalsCustomerService-usa@elsevier.com **(for print support) and** JournalsOnlineSupport-usa@elsevier.com **(for online support).**

Reprints. For copies of 100 or more of articles in this publication, please contact the Commercial Reprints Department, Elsevier Inc., 360 Park Avenue South, New York, New York, 10010-1710; Tel.: 212-633-3874, Fax: 212-633-3820, and E-mail: reprints@elsevier.com.

Critical Care Nursing Clinics of North America is covered in *MEDLINE/PubMed (Index Medicus), International Nursing Index, Nursing Citation Index, Cumulative Index to Nursing and Allied Health Literature,* and *RNdex Top 100.*

Contributors

CONSULTING EDITOR

JAN FOSTER, PhD, APRN, CNS
Formerly, Associate Professor, College of Nursing, Texas Woman's University, Houston, Texas; Currently, President, Nursing Inquiry and Intervention, Inc, The Woodlands, Texas

EDITOR

DEBORAH W. CHAPA, PhD, ACNP-BC, ACHPN, FAANP
Nurse Practitioner, Lee Palliative Care, Lee Health, Fort Myers, Florida

AUTHORS

BIMBOLA FOLA AKINTADE, PhD, MBA, MHA, CCRN, ACNP-BC, NEA-BC
University of Maryland School of Nursing, Baltimore, Maryland

MARY-MICHAEL BROWN, DNP, RN, CENP
Vice President, Nursing Practice Innovation, MedStar Health, Columbia, Maryland

STACEY G. BROWNING, DNP, MSN, RN
Assistant Professor, School of Nursing, College of Behavioral and Health Sciences, Middle Tennessee State University, Murfreesboro, Tennessee

SHARON E. BRYANT, DNP, ACNP-BC, RN, MSN
Assistant Professor of Nursing, Vanderbilt University School of Nursing, Nashville, Tennessee

DEBORAH W. CHAPA, PhD, ACNP-BC, ACHPN, FAANP
Nurse Practitioner, Lee Palliative Care, Lee Health, Fort Myers, Florida

SAREEN GROPPER, PhD-Nutrition, RDN, LDN
Professor, Christine E. Lynn College of Nursing, Florida Atlantic University, Boca Raton, Florida

DENNIS HUNT, EdD, CSCS
Assistant Professor, Florida Gulf Coast University, Fort Myers, Florida

ISLANDE JOSEPH, BSN, RN
Medical Intensive Care Unit, Lee Memorial Hospital, Fort Myers, Florida

CAITLIN LACH, BSN, RN
College of Nursing, University of Florida, Shands Children's Hospital, Gainesville, Florida

RENEE McCAULEY, MSN, RN, CCRN
Medical Intensive Care Unit, Lee Memorial Hospital, Fort Myers, Florida

MOLLY E. McGETRICK, MD
Critical Care Fellow, Division of Pediatric Critical Care, The University of Texas Southwestern Medical Center, Dallas, Texas; Division of Pediatrics, University of Florida, Gainesville, Florida

KATHRYN McNABB, DNP, AGACNP, RN, MSN
Instructor of Nursing, Vanderbilt University School of Nursing, Nashville, Tennessee

CRYSTAL L. MORALES, MS, BSN, RN
Director, High Reliability and Safety, MedStar Institute for Quality and Safety, Washington, DC

ANGELA MOREHEAD, DNP, FNP-BC, RN
Assistant Professor, Nursing, Middle Tennessee State University, Murfreesboro, Tennessee

JODI E. MULLEN, RN-BC
University of Florida, Shands Children's Hospital, Gainesville, Florida

JENNIFER C. MUNOZ-PAREJA, MD
Associate Professor, Division of Pediatric Critical Care, Department of Pediatrics, University of Florida, Gainesville, Florida

KATHARINE OUTEN, DNP, AGACNP-BC, AGCNS-BC
University of Maryland Medical Center, Baltimore, Maryland

LYNN C. PARSONS, PhD, MSN, RN, NEA-BC
Center for Health, Education and Research, Morehead State University, Morehead, Kentucky

GARRETT SALMON, DNP, MS, BSN, APRN, CRNA
Assistant Professor, Nursing, Middle Tennessee State University, Murfreesboro, Tennessee

MICHELE A. WALTERS, DNP, APRN, FNP-BC
St. Claire Family Medicine Express, Morehead State University, Morehead, Kentucky

DOROTHY WHOLIHAN, DNP, AGPCNP-BC, GNP-BC, ACHPN, FPCN
Clinical Associate Professor, Director of Palliative Care NP Specialty Program, NYU Rory Meyers College of Nursing, New York, New York

Contents

Critical care clinicians involved serious adverse events may experience a
constellation of distressing emotions that may interfere with home and
work life. Offering support after a serious adverse event may restore a clinician's ability to cope with the event, reestablish emotional balance and
assist a clinician to function capably in the workplace and at home. A
description of a care for the caregiver program implementation at a 10-
hospital health system provides a roadmap to implement this program in
other hospitals and health systems.

Several hospital interventions increase patient risk for developing delirium,
including mechanical ventilation, monitoring devices, medication interactions, urinary catheters, interrupted sleep cycles, and use of physical restraints. Developing delirium leads to increased length of hospital stay,
likelihood of requiring long-term care services after discharge, and risk
of mortality following hospitalization. Longer periods of delirium worsen
cognition, executive functioning, ability to complete activities of daily
living, and sensorimotor functioning. Routine screening and early recognition prevent or reduce the long-term health and financial effects of
delirium. The Confusion Assessment Method is a useable tool for
screening noncritically ill adult patients for delirium.

Delirium is a common disease process in the pediatric critical care unit, yet
practices for screening and prevention vary drastically between institutions. The authors hypothesized that surveying pediatric residents and
nurses who care for patients in the intensive care setting would expose
misunderstandings about delirium. They brought to light common incorrect beliefs that benzodiazepines are appropriate therapy for delirium
and that children who are delirious will not have memories of the experience. Many nurses and residents listed that they were not comfortable
or were extremely uncomfortable identifying delirious patients. Findings
demonstrate an opportunity to improve on nursing and resident
knowledge.

Multiple evaluation tools exist, and the core components of the theoretic burnout tools are vague and ambiguous and overlap legitimate mental health diseases, such as depression. Applied therapeutic interventions support decreased perceived burnout and staff turnover and improved overall well-being of nurses. Research postulates that decreased levels of burnout are associated with improved quality of patient care, communication, and trust, combined with decreases in patient morbidity and mortality, and ultimately, a decrease in the overall financial cost of care.

CRITICAL CARE NURSING
CLINICS OF NORTH AMERICA

SERIES OF RELATED INTEREST

Nursing Clinics of North America
http://www.nursing.theclinics.com

THE CLINICS ARE AVAILABLE ONLINE!
Access your subscription at:
www.theclinics.com

Preface

Improvement of Psychosocial Outcomes in Patients with Critical Care Illness Positively Impacts Outcomes for Patients and Caregivers

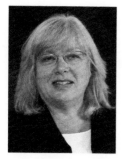

Deborah W. Chapa, PhD, ACNP-BC, ACHPN, FAANP
Editor

Psychosocial issues in patients and families impact outcomes for patients who have critical illness. In the United States, it has been estimated that $3500 per day is spent on critical care admissions and may account for 13% of hospital costs. Half of all people in the United States may spend time in critical care during their final year of life. There is a new condition arising termed chronic critical illness. Children who spend time in critical care may be at risk for long-term psychosocial disadvantage. Psychosocial issues, such as delirium, anxiety, posttraumatic stress disorder, depression, posttraumatic stress disorder, and postintensive care syndrome, significantly impact patients and caregivers. Patients also experience psychosocial trauma when moving from intensive care to palliative care.

It is imperative that those caring for patients in the intensive care setting understand the impact, diagnosis, and management strategies of psychosocial issues for patients and caregivers. Caregivers include families and all members of the interdisciplinary team. If we do not properly address these issues, patients are at risk for increased mortality, decreased functional status, and decreased quality of life. Caregivers are at risk for depression, burnout, anxiety, and posttraumatic stress disorder. Nurses play a vital

Crit Care Nurs Clin N Am 31 (2019) ix–x
https://doi.org/10.1016/j.cnc.2019.09.001
0899-5885/19/© 2019 Published by Elsevier Inc.

role in diagnosis and interventions to promote positive psychosocial outcomes for patients, caregivers, and themselves.

Deborah W. Chapa, PhD, ACNP-BC, ACHPN, FAANP
Lee Palliative Care
8925 Colonial Center Drive
Building A Suite 1000
Fort Myers, FL 33905, USA

E-mail address:
Deborah.Chapa@leehealth.org

Creating a Care for the Caregiver Program in a Ten-Hospital Health System

Crystal L. Morales, MS, BSN, RN[a], Mary-Michael Brown, DNP, RN, CENP[b],*

KEYWORDS

- Second victim • Care for the caregiver • Adverse event
- Communication and optimal resolution

KEY POINTS

- Serious adverse events can occur in the critical care setting owing to the acuity of patients and its fast-paced and continuously changing environment.
- The emotional aftermath of being involved in a serious adverse event can interfere with a clinicians' home and work life.
- Developing a care for the caregiver program using an established program and materials can be restorative to clinicians involved in serious adverse events.

INTRODUCTION

To the uninitiated, a critical care unit can be a chaotic environment[1,2] filled with unfamiliar equipment, sounds, and activities, along with clinicians who may use unrecognizable words or acronyms. Over time, critical care clinicians acclimate to this environment and regularly manage the crises associated with caring for the sickest patients in a hospital. Continuously adjusting to this fast-paced and frenetic environment can take its toll on clinicians by precipitating stress,[3–6] burnout,[7,8] compassion fatigue,[9] and moral distress.[1,10]

The American Association of Critical Care Nurses' Healthy Work Environment Standards promote safe, healing, and humane work and care environments that can potentially prevent or mitigate the extent of these negative conditions.[11] However, full implementation of these standards has not yet been achieved and unhealthy work environments may persist.[11] Consequently, when an unanticipated adverse event occurs that may have been precipitated by a clinician's error, or

Disclosure Statement: No disclosures. The authors have nothing to disclose.
[a] High Reliability and Safety, Medstar Institute for Quality and Safety, 3007 Tilden Street, Northwest, Suite 5N, Washington, DC 20008, USA; [b] Nursing Practice Innovation, Medstar Health, 10980 Grantchester Place, 6101, Columbia, MD 21044, USA
* Corresponding author.
E-mail address: mary-michael.brown@medstar.net

Crit Care Nurs Clin N Am 31 (2019) 461–473
https://doi.org/10.1016/j.cnc.2019.07.001
0899-5885/19/© 2019 Elsevier Inc. All rights reserved.

when clinicians are exposed to other traumatic situations, a safe, healing, and humane environment in which to contend with these upsetting or unsettling events may be unavailable. The ensuing turmoil may test the limits of a clinician's emotional and physical resilience and may impede the clinician's ability to continue to care for his or her patients in his or her customary skilled and compassionate fashion.

We describe the development of a system-wide program to support clinicians when their actions may have catalyzed a serious, unintended, adverse patient outcome or when clinicians themselves have experienced a highly emotional and impressionable event. This care for the caregiver program is considered in detail and recommendations are offered to implement a similar program in other critical care units, hospitals, and health systems.

HUMAN RESPONSES TO SERIOUS UNINTENDED EVENTS

Critical care clinicians regularly care for patients who are suffering from pain, life-threatening injuries, life-limiting conditions, and devastating complications, the latter of which may be completely unanticipated. Communication issues may surface with patients' families and other health care providers[2] and anxious family members may interfere with[12] or challenge clinicians' decisions. Interprofessional disagreements about the plan of care may surface. Rotating night shift work and extended working hours may compound these situations,[13] as may staff shortages.[14]

In their discussion about critical incidents, or those serious unanticipated adverse events that extract a deeply emotional reaction, de Boer and her colleagues[15] describe critical care nurses' potential coping responses to these incidents. Reflecting on or talking about the event illustrates active, problem-solving coping.[15] This approach includes revisiting and thinking through the event, discussing the event with others, and conducting reality testing.[15] Using problem-solving coping can potentially expedite recovery from the critical event.

Conversely, denying, minimizing, or suppressing the event marks defensive coping.[15] Defensive coping may include rationalizing the event or withdrawing from or dissociating oneself from the event.[15] Although defensive coping may help the individual clinician in the short run, this approach can result in repetitive thoughts or recurring dreams about the incident and, if unresolved, can potentially result in symptoms of posttraumatic stress disorder.[15]

When an unanticipated serious, adverse event is a result of human error, such as a fatal medication mistake, the involved clinicians may experience disbelief, disgrace, dread, or distress as they blame themselves or when others blame them for the event. Davidson and her colleagues[16] explored the conditions of moral distress and blame-related distress resulting from a negative patient outcome by surveying 157 oncology and critical care clinicians about their experiences with these conditions in their workplace. The authors distinguished moral distress, which prevents a clinician from taking action, with blame-related distress, which emerges after a clinician has taken action.[16] More than three-fourths of survey respondents acknowledged experiencing moral distress and one-half of survey respondents described being blamed for a negative patient outcome.[16] The majority of surveyed participants cited coworkers, family, and friends as their primary resources to process their experiences.[16] Davidson and colleagues[16] point out that these preferences mirror those of individuals reacting to an event that resulted in a negative patient outcome, so-called second victims.[17–19]

SECOND VICTIMS

Historically, clinicians involved in a serious unintended negative patient outcome may have suffered in silence, particularly if emotional support was unavailable or insufficient. Clinicians may experience guilt, shame,[20] and embarrassment, and lack the confidence to return to work following the event.[17] In 2000, Wu coined the term second victim to identify clinicians involved in a mistake that led to patient harm and who were without the resources to help process and grieve effectively about the error.[21] The events surrounding the 10-fold overdose made by nurse Kimberly Hiatt and her subsequent suicide is a heartbreaking and extreme example of the continuum of emotions faced, and actions taken by, a second victim.[22]

In 2009, Scott and her associates[17] at the University of Missouri Health System reported the results of semistructured interviews with 31 second victims who were involved in adverse patient events. The authors noted that these clinicians subsequently experienced a variety of physical and psychosocial symptoms after being involved in an adverse event that led to patient harm and described 6 predictable stages of recovery: chaos and accident response, intrusive reflections, restoring personal integrity, enduring the inquisition, obtaining emotional first aid, and moving on.[17]

Chaos and Accident Response

When the adverse event was recognized, the second victims described the ensuing chaos as multiple activities occurring simultaneously.[17] These included applying life-sustaining measures while discerning what, how, and why the event just happened.[17] As involved clinicians responded to the event, they noted becoming unfocused as they considered their role in the occurrence and criticized themselves when they needed to enlist the help of a peer to manage the situation owing to their unfocused state.[17]

Intrusive Reflections

After the event occurred, Scott and her colleagues[17] reported that second victims reenacted the event in their minds and expressed self-doubt or second-guessed their actions. Intrusive reflections were characterized by repeatedly asking "what if" questions and resulted in temporary loss of confidence.[17(p327)]

Restoring Personal Integrity

As second victims attempted to restore their personal integrity, they reported seeking solace from a trusted individual, who could be a work associate, supervisor, family member, or friend.[17] Other second victims described not knowing to whom they could turn for support because they considered it unlikely that another individual could fully appreciate the event and the extent of the personal toll it extracted.[17] Further, second victims reported the distressing personal consequences when met with unsupportive or negative reactions by colleagues, which deepened self-doubt, further degraded self-confidence, and impeded return of their sense of personal integrity.[17]

Enduring the Inquisition

After the event occurred, second victims described the aftermath of the event when realizing an institutional investigation would follow.[17] Second victims became concerned about job loss, license revocation, and possible litigation. Other second victims reported feelings of isolation when they became uncertain with whom they could discuss the events based on unclear interpretations of the Health Insurance Portability and Accountability Act.[17]

Obtaining Emotional First Aid

Scott and colleagues[17] noted that second victims sought emotional support in multiple ways yet described the limitations inherent in these means. Some second victims again worried about to whom they could speak based on potential violations of the Health Insurance Portability and Accountability Act or that no one could fully understand the depth of their experience.[17]

Moving on: Dropping Out, Surviving, or Thriving

The second victims in the study by Scott and colleagues[17] conveyed difficulty with overcoming the event, including forgiving themselves for the event. Some second victims chose to change their department or leave their jobs or their profession; others voiced an inability to move past the event and continued to ruminate about it.[17] Some second victims remained cognizant of the event, shared their experience with colleagues, spoke openly about their experience, and changed their clinical practices to prevent the future occurrence of similar events.[17]

Building on the interviews with the 31 second victims originally studied, Scott and her colleagues[18] described the development and deployment of a rapid response team for second victims called the Scott Three-Tiered Integrated Model of Interventional Support. This program, which was available 24 hours a day, 7 days a week in University of Missouri hospitals, consisted of specially trained peers who formed the 3-tier response team. Tier 1 offered first responder support in which a team peer triaged the situation. This involved asking the second victims if they were "okay" and providing emotional first aid as needed and requested.[18(p236)] The authors noted that approximately 60% of second victims found tier 1 support adequate.[18]

Tier 2 attention included continuing support for the individuals who were identified as a second victim in an earlier situation.[18] Trained peer supporters within high-risk areas observed their colleagues for signs and symptoms of second victim characteristics as the event investigation continued.[18] When indicated, the trained peer supporters became rapid responders by referring second victims to other resources, such as contact with safety experts or risk managers.[18] Scott and her associates[18] acknowledged the additional training and important roles tier 2 peer supporters presented during team debriefings after the event. The authors estimated that about 30% of second victims benefitted from tier 2 support.[18]

Tier 3 provided rapid access to professional counseling for second victims whose emotional needs could not be met by members of the peer rapid response team through tier 1 or tier 2 actions.[18] Resources offered in a tier 3 response included referrals to a chaplain, social worker, employee assistance personnel, or psychologists.[18]

COMMUNICATION AND OPTIMAL RESOLUTION

Ideally, identifying and supporting second victims is part of a larger program of adverse patient event management that includes disclosing unanticipated adverse events to patients and their families and preemptively offering an apology, explanation, corrective action plan, and potential restitution for the events.[23] Driven by malpractice reform, these communication and resolution programs (CRP) were first attributed to the Lexington Veteran's Affairs hospital in 1987, and subsequently received endorsement by the Joint Commission in 2001, when limited disclosure of adverse patient events was initiated as part of the accreditation process.[24] These efforts were followed by the introduction of CRPs in University of Michigan and several US academic medical centers.[24] In 2009, President Obama commissioned the

Agency for Healthcare Research and Quality (AHRQ) to fund CRP demonstration projects to evaluate their influence on patient safety and potential malpractice lawsuits.[24]

In 2012, several new safety initiatives were started within our health system. First, a system vice president for quality and safety was hired who had direct, personal experience with the Seven Pillar Program at University of Illinois Medical Center at Chicago.[25] This program combined CRP tenets with clinician education and training.[25] Second, under the direction of the system vice president for quality and safety, our 10-hospital health system designed and initiated a high reliability organization roadmap that incorporated process designs, a fair and just culture, human factors engineering, patient and family partnerships, and transparency about adverse patient events. Third, owing to our health system's renewed commitment to patient safety, in 2013 our health system participated in a 24-month collaborative with 2 other health systems to implement the AHRQ's Communication and Optimal Resolution (CANDOR) toolkit.[26] The goal of the CANDOR project was to create a comprehensive medical liability toolkit, test the tools in practice, determine the feasibility of implementing the toolkit, and ascertain its effectiveness. The toolkit leveraged all elements of a CRP through 8 training modules, PowerPoint slide decks, facilitator notes, and other tools (**Box 1**).[26] Our health system's contribution to the CANDOR toolkit was the creation of a comprehensive event review process; however, we fully implemented the entire CANDOR program in all 10 hospitals. Key to implementing the CANDOR process was building a "Go Team" to respond to serious unanticipated events.

THE GO TEAM

When a serious, unanticipated event occurs in one of our hospitals, the CANDOR process is now activated through a Go Team. This team, which is an amalgam of the National Transportation Safety Board Go Team[27] and components of the Scott Three-Tiered Integrated Model of Interventional Support,[18] consists of CANDOR-trained peers including nurses, physicians, chaplains, risk managers, and safety champions. When a serious unanticipated adverse event occurs, Go Team members provide the following services: patient communication consultation services, care for the caregiver, and event review initiation.

When receiving notification of the event, Go Team members that serve as part of the patient communication consultation services arrive and support or coach involved individuals on how to respond to patients and family members in a timely, empathetic, consistent, and patient-centered way. Risk manager Go

---

Box 1
CANDOR modules

Module 1	An overview of the CANDOR process
Module 2	Obtaining organizational buy-in and support
Module 3	Preparing for implementation: gap analysis
Module 4	Event reporting, event investigation and analysis
Module 5	Response and disclosure
Module 6	Care for the Caregiver program implementation guide
Module 7	Resolution
Module 8	Organizational learning and sustainability

Data from Agency for Healthcare Research and Quality. Communication and optimal resolution (CANDOR) toolkit. Content last reviewed September 2017. http://www.ahrq.gov/professionals/quality-patient-safety/patient-safety-resources/resources/candor/introduction.html. Accessed February 28, 2019.

Team members may provide immediate financial respite to affected patients and families by suspending hospital bills or offering other forms of financial assistance, such as absorbing travel or hotel costs for family members. The network of CANDOR-trained peers offers support for anyone involved in the serious unanticipated event.

Care for the caregiver may be activated to provide immediate emotional first aid to care team associates affected by an event. Short-term and long-term needs of the affected caregivers are determined during these encounters.

Teams of individuals who have been trained to conduct a timely, objective and thorough analysis of the serious unanticipated adverse event do so using a systems-based approach. This event review considers factors that may have contributed to the event, such as the availability of functional equipment, workflow processes, staffing, and policies and procedures. Importantly, the emphasis is not on who made an error, but rather gaining insight into how clinicians made decisions in that instance is sought to discover how systems issues and processes may have contributed to the event. Sustainable solutions and lessons learned for other clinicians are gathered from the event review and disseminated across our health system through a weekly serious safety event email or by developing and dispatching a safety alert communication from our health system executive team. Individual clinicians may spread awareness by choosing to use the event at daily inpatient safety huddles or as a safety moment at the beginning of a meeting or conference call.

BUILDING THE CARE FOR THE CAREGIVER PROGRAM

A key part of the AHRQ CANDOR collaborative was the development and implementation of our care for the caregiver program, which received the direct support and guidance of Dr Susan Scott, who served as faculty for our institutional training. Owing to the size of our 10-hospital health system, a train-the-trainer approach was selected to build a team of instructors to expediently establish the CANDOR program and our care for the caregiver program across all 10 of our hospitals. The first step in this process was to select points of contact from all 10 hospitals to serve as the care for the caregiver lead at their respective entities. Senior hospital leaders in each entity identified individuals in their organization who demonstrated exceptional communication skills, high emotional intelligence, and leadership acumen to serve as care for the caregiver leads. Once these points of contact were identified, they were invited to participate in a 1-hour, in-person introductory care for the caregiver workshop that centered on 5 objectives (**Box 2**). These objectives were

---

Box 2
Objectives of the introductory care-for-the-caregiver session

Objective 1	Discuss why care for the caregiver is needed.
Objective 2	Describe the second victim trajectory.
Objective 3	Identify support strategy model and interventions
Objective 4	Describe how to provide peer support.
Objective 5	Demonstrate the use of the care for the caregiver support program planning tool.

Data from Agency for Healthcare Research and Quality. Communication and optimal resolution (CANDOR) toolkit. Content last reviewed September 2017. http://www.ahrq.gov/professionals/quality-patient-safety/patient-safety-resources/resources/candor/introduction.html. Accessed February 28, 2019.

addressed using didactic instruction that included real examples of serious unintended adverse event scenarios in an open lecture style environment where the learners where encouraged to ask questions and discuss methods to approach and manage the training scenarios.

After the initial training, the next step was for the local program leaders to begin to assemble a local team of peer supporters who would provide the care for the caregiver services. Under the direct tutelage of Dr Susan Scott, our local program leaders were selected from chaplains, palliative care team members, social workers, occupational health workers, and members from the employee assistance program. Other team members included nurse leaders, physicians, pharmacists, and educators, who rounded out the multidisciplinary care for the caregiver team. Training sessions for care for the caregiver team members were held at all 10 hospitals and introduced peer support concepts and set overall expectations of team members. Owing to the size and unique infrastructure of each of our entities, hospital care for the caregiver team leaders were offered the latitude of determining the size and functional operation of their respective teams.

Each member of the care for the caregiver team brings a unique perspective to the team based on his or her diverse role and experience. This distinctive outlook is augmented by the size, type, and clinical services offered at each of our hospital. This diversity is embraced and leveraged to provide personalized emotional support to involved clinicians, triage the direct caregiver's emotional needs, and marshal additional resources, should the caregiver need them. Care for the caregiver services are confidential and are not intended to investigate or reexamine the event, but rather to ascertain how the involved clinician is feeling and contending with the emotions associated with the event. All individuals have the right to accept or decline the care for the caregiver services. It is worth noting here that, although the care for the caregiver program originally was established to respond to a patient harm event, as our experience and recognition accumulate, the program since has evolved and expanded to responding to other events such as divorce, loss of a loved one, burnout, and domestic abuse.

NOTIFICATION AND DEPLOYMENT OF CARE FOR THE CAREGIVER

During CANDOR implementation training, Go Teams defined how the care for the caregiver teams would be notified and deployed. To ensure widespread, uncomplicated access to the program, we established more than one means of peer support contact. These means included paging, emailing, texting, or telephoning a member of the care for the caregiver team. Brochures describing care for the caregiver services were created to market the program and were placed strategically in areas where high numbers of associates would see them. The brochures introduced the program and displayed information on how to contact the team for peer support. It is important to note that anyone can request care for the caregiver services either on one's own behalf or on behalf of another individual.

All of our hospital associates use an electronic patient safety event management system (PSEMS) to record details of serious unintended adverse events, near-misses, and "good catch" events. A unique data field was created in the PSEMS that allows our associates, who manage and review these events, to request care for the caregiver services for those involved in a serious unanticipated adverse event at the same time they are reviewing the PSEMS file (**Fig. 1**). Further, a unique data field will be added in the near future that will permit authors of the PSEMS file to request care for the caregiver services. This data field is positioned strategically near the

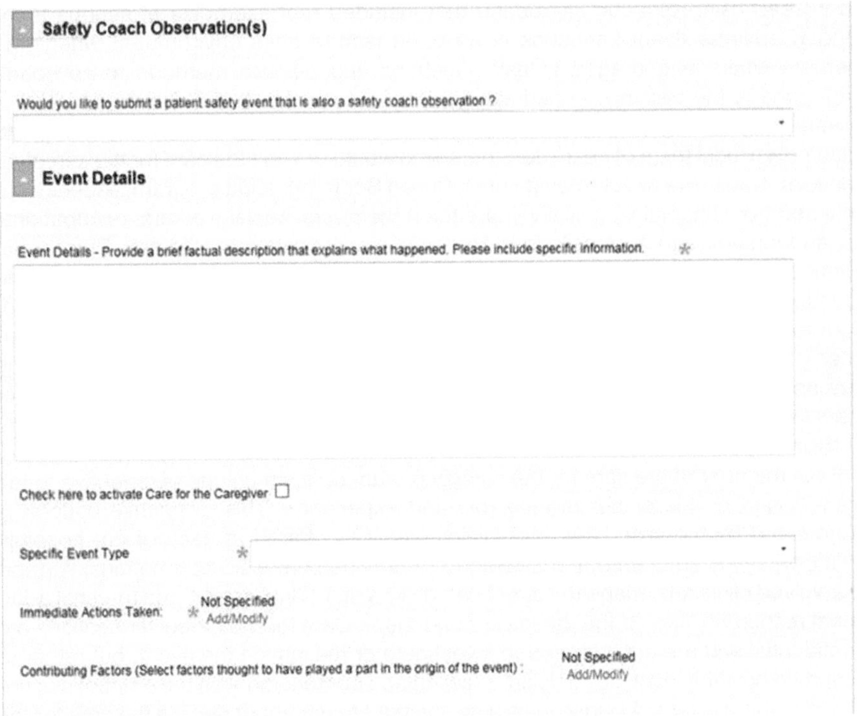
Safety Coach Observation(s)

Would you like to submit a patient safety event that is also a safety coach observation ?

Event Details

Event Details - Provide a brief factual description that explains what happened. Please include specific information. *

Check here to activate Care for the Caregiver ☐

Specific Event Type *

Immediate Actions Taken: * Not Specified Add/Modify

Contributing Factors (Select factors thought to have played a part in the origin of the event) : Not Specified Add/Modify

Fig. 1. HeRO (MedStar Health, Columbia, MD) PSEMS file entry with care for the caregiver check box.

narrative data entry area to promote visibility of the service as the author completes a description of the event. Once the care for the caregiver service is selected, the individual assigned to receive those specific alerts at that particular hospital receives an email notification that a request for care for the caregiver has been made. Upon receiving a request for care for the caregiver services, that individual will determine which Go Team member is best suited to approach the individual in need. These decisions are based on the type of event and the individual(s) involved.

Our goal for the initial encounter is to provide peer-to-peer support. Once a decision has been made as to who is going to provide support, that individual will either connect with that individual's direct supervisor to find a mutually convenient time to meet in person or reach out to that individual directly to arrange a time either to talk by telephone or meet in person. During the initial in-person encounter, the individual receiving services is greeted with a "Thinking of You" bag that contains a journal, dark chocolate, a stress ball, and tissues. We have found that this small token helps to build rapport and lets the individual know how much he or she is valued as a member of the hospital team. Care for the caregiver has become ingrained in our health system's culture and workflow around serious unanticipated outcomes. Currently, when any of our health system safety associates and Go Team members are notified of a serious unanticipated outcome, one of the first questions asked is, "Has care for the caregiver been offered?"

The success and growth of this program is due largely to the local and system-level leadership support it received and continues to receive. Early in the inception of the care for the caregiver program, Sorrell King, author of *Josie's Story*,[28] founder of the Josie King Foundation, and an active member of our health system's Patient and Family Advisory Council, reached out and recognized our work. Ms King's 18-month-old daughter, Josie, died as a result of severe dehydration, undetected sepsis, and a narcotic-related medication error when Josie was hospitalized with a burn injury. Ms King supported our efforts by providing 100 Josie King nursing journals to distribute during our care for the caregiver encounters. Presently, more than 2500 "Thinking of You" bags have been provided through our care for the caregiver program across our 10 hospitals. The following scenarios offer insight into the process and outcomes of our care for the caregiver program.

CARE FOR THE CAREGIVER SCENARIOS
Scenario 1: Care for a Critical Care Intensivist

A new critical care intensivist was caring for a patient who suffered from morbid obesity, altered mental status, pulmonary edema, and pneumonia, the latter of which required mechanical ventilation. During intubation, the team used soft wrist restraints for airway protection while sedation was achieved. Despite these safety efforts, the patient self-extubated the endotracheal tube. The critical care team immediately responded; however, despite multiple attempts, the intensivist was unable to reintubate the patient. Knowing that the patient required mechanical ventilation, an emergent bedside cricothryrotomy was performed with the assistance of the anesthesia team. The patient was then taken immediately to the operating room for a tracheostomy. The patient returned to the critical care unit in stable condition.

The intensivist who performed the emergent bedside cricothyrotomy was visibly shaken after the procedure. Appreciating how disturbing this event had been for the intensivist, the critical care unit director contacted the lead of the care for the caregiver team to request support for this intensivist. The critical care unit director recognized that the involved intensivist was both new to the critical care team that this was the first time this intensivist had performed an emergent bedside cricothryrotomy. A member of the care for the caregiver team arrived in the critical care unit with a "Thinking of You" bag to check in with the intensivist and to let her know that everyone recognized how well she had performed in an unexpectedly difficult situation. In turn, the intensivist expressed gratitude for the support from both the critical care unit staff and the care for the caregiver program.

Scenario 2: Care for a Critical Care Nurse

A 34-year-old patient with a history of ulcerative colitis presented to the emergency department with complaints of abdominal pain, bloody stools, and general malaise for the past week. The patient was hypotensive, febrile, and tachycardic upon arrival. The patient was quickly diagnosed with sepsis related to toxic megacolon with perforation and was intubated, started on fluid resuscitation, antibiotics, vasopressive medications and was admitted to the intensive care unit (ICU). Upon arrival to the ICU, the intensivist spoke with the patient's husband and described the severity of the patient's condition and her poor prognosis. The patient's husband stated that he understood his wife's grave condition and asked that all measures be used to save his wife's life particularly because they had 2 small children at home that very much needed their mother.

Over the next 2 days, the patient's husband stayed at her bedside and family members would bring the children in to the ICU to visit with their mother. The critical care nurses created diversionary activities for them and made every attempt to make the visits as meaningful and pleasant as possible. The critical care nurses often cried after the family left because they were deeply saddened by the inability to change, fix, or heal this patient. They also expressed how emotionally exhausting it was to observe the poignant yet limited interactions between the fully sedated, unconscious patient and her children. Many of the nurses in the ICU had children the same age and were deeply influenced by this family's experience. Despite aggressive interventions, the patient's condition continued to deteriorate. The patient subsequently died 3 days after being admitted to the ICU, with her husband, children, and other family members at her bedside. It was a somber day.

Although deaths in the ICU can have an impact on the staff, this patient's death was particularly difficult. The nursing director reached out to the care for the caregiver lead and arranged for several group sessions to connect with all the nurses in the ICU. The sessions were tearful and extended beyond the 1-hour scheduled session. In addition to these on-site care for the caregiver sessions, several critical care nurses were referred and accepted employee assistance program consultation. The nurses receiving care for the caregiver described feeling grateful for the opportunity to talk openly without judgment about how this event was impacting them. These sessions also enabled peer support among the critical care nursing team.

REFLECTIONS AND LESSONS LEARNED

When reflecting on the genesis and evolution of our care for the caregiver program, we recognize that our approach has similarities and differences when compared with other peer support initiatives. One distinction is how members of the care for the caregiver team were and are currently selected. Not unlike the process used by Lane and colleagues[20] and Scott and colleagues,[18] we invited entity leaders to suggest individuals or we sought out certain professionals, such as chaplains or social workers, to serve as peer supporters. The approach that Graham and her colleagues[29] describe, which is asking peers to nominate other peers to whom they turn for peer support as potential members of a caregiver support team, offers a compelling and different approach for member selection. It has prompted us to consider how we will recruit and revitalize our care for the caregiver teams after member turnover. Reflecting on Denham's 5 rights of second victims, which are just treatment, respect, understanding and compassion, supportive care, and transparency,[30] has reenergized our efforts to be more intentional in recognizing opportunities to learn from second victims and create venues for both support and system learning. Last, nurses comprise the top volume professional requesting care for the caregiver services, which correlates with their distinction as the top volume authors of PSEMS files. Among nurses and others, there is an array of reasons for the care for the caregiver requests, the majority of which involve a patient-related event. This finding underscores our resolve to extend care for the caregiver services universally to all associates and reinvigorate our efforts to market this valuable program.

We offer several lessons learned for other critical care units, hospitals, and health systems that are interested in building and deploying a care for the caregiver program. First, the care for the caregiver team requires unwavering executive support. This includes support for the resources required to (a) initiate and provide ongoing train-the-trainer sessions using the CANDOR toolkit, (b) create the infrastructure to dispatch care for the caregiver team members when needed, (c) reconstitute the care for the caregiver team after team member turnover, and (d) intentionally hardwire the program and processes. Second, establishing a means to track and trend care for the caregiver services offered, including types of professionals involved, types of events, high-volume units, duration of care for the caregiver encounter, and recipient responses to the encounter are critical. These data assist us with the future evolution of our program, including content to emphasize in general education about care for the caregiver services and curriculum for our annual care for the caregiver retreat. Third, it is important to establish regularly scheduled, in-person or virtual meetings with care for the caregiver team members to debrief on care for the caregiver instances and exchange local or unique approaches that have been successful and well-received. Fourth, the use of all available resources in the AHRQ CANDOR toolkit enhances the care for the caregiver program.

Future directions in our journey to provide care for the caregiver services to our colleagues include adding simulation training to the current train-the-trainer program, expanding the care for the caregiver program to the ambulatory arena as well as considering the feasibility of conducting a cost-benefit analysis of the program as described by Endrees and colleagues.[31] For our critical care nursing colleagues specifically, framing a care for the caregiver program using the AACN healthy work environment standards may offer insight into the synergy between our program and these standards.[32]

SUMMARY

Owing to the chaotic and stressful nature of the critical care environment, critical care nurses and other clinicians are at risk for involvement in or exposure to conditions leading to unexpected, adverse patient outcomes and events. A care for the caregiver program is a means to support our care team members in particularly stressful situations or when care does not go as planned. When our associates feel safe and supported, we advance our high reliability journey and ultimately the quality of care that our patients receive.

REFERENCES

1. Huffman DM, Rittenmeyer L. How professional nurses working in hospital environments experience moral distress: a systematic review. Crit Care Nurs Clin North Am 2012;24(1):91–100.
2. Levy MM. Caring for the caregiver. Crit Care Clin 2004;20(3):541–7.
3. Baid H. Resilience in critical care nurses. Nurs Crit Care 2018;23(6):281–2.
4. Burgess L, Irvine F, Walllymahmed A. Personality, stress and coping in intensive care nurses: a descriptive exploratory study. Nurs Crit Care 2016;15(3):129–40.
5. Kapoor S, Morgan CK, Siddique MA, et al. "Sacred pause" in the ICU: evaluation of a ritual and intervention to lower distress and burnout. Am J Hosp Palliat Care 2018;35(10):1337–41.
6. Mealer M, Hodapp R, Conrad D, et al. Designing a resilience program for critical care nurses. AACN Adv Crit Care 2017;28(4):359–65.
7. Moss M, Good VS, Gorzal D, et al. An official critical care societies collaborative statement: burnout syndrome in critical care healthcare professionals: a call to action. Chest 2016;150(1):17–26.
8. Papathanassoglou E, Karanikola M. Stress in critical care: a policy perspective. Nurs Crit Care 2018;23(3):117–20.
9. Kelly LA, Lefton C. Effect of meaningful recognition on critical care nurses' compassion fatigue. Am J Crit Care 2017;26(6):438–44.
10. McAndrew NS, Leske J, Schroeter K. Moral distress in critical care nursing: the state science. Nurs Ethics 2018;25(5):552–70.

11. Barden C, Cassidy L, Cardin S. AACN Standards for Establishing and Sustaining Healthy Work Environments: A Journey to Excellence. 2nd edition. Aliso Viejo (CA): American Association of Critical-Care Nurses; 2016.

12. Carlson EB, Spain DA, Muhtadie L, et al. Care and caring in the ICU: family members distress and perceptions about staff skills, communication, and emotional support. J Crit Care 2015;30(3):557–61.

13. Jarden RJ, Sandham M, Siegert RJ, et al. Strengthening workplace well-being: perceptions of intensive care nurses. Nurs Crit Care 2019;24(1):15–23.

14. Davidson JE, Agan DL, Chakedis S, et al. Workplace blame and related concepts: an analysis of three case studies. Chest 2015;148(2):543–9.

15. de Boer J, van Rikxoort S, Bakker AB, et al. Critical incidents among intensive care unit nurses and their need for support: explorative interviews. Nurs Crit Care 2014;19(4):166–74.

16. Davidson JE, Agan DL, Chakedis S. Exploring distress caused by blame for a negative patient outcome. J Nurs Adm 2016;46(1):18–24.

17. Scott SD, Hirschinger LE, Cox KR, et al. The natural history of recovery for the healthcare provider "second victim" after adverse patient events. Qual Saf Health Care 2009;18(5):325–30.

18. Scott SD, Hirschinger LI, Cox KR, et al. Caring for our own: deploying a system-wide second victim rapid response team. Jt Comm J Qual Patient Saf 2010;36(5): 233–40.

19. Seys D, Scott S, Wu A, et al. Supporting involved health care professionals (second victims) following an adverse health event: a literature review. Int J Nurs Stud 2013;50(5):678–87.

20. Lane MA, Newman BM, Taylor MZ, et al. Supporting clinicians after adverse events: development of a clinician peer support program. J Patient Saf 2018; 14(3):e56–60.

21. Wu AW. Medical error: the second victim. BMJ 2000;320(7237):726.

22. Ostrom CM. Nurses suicide follows tragedy. Seattle Times 2011. Available at: https://www.seattletimes.com/seattle-news/nurses-suicide-follows-tragedy/. Accessed February 28, 2019.

23. Mello MM, Boothman RC, McDonald T, et al. Communication-and-resolution programs: the challenges and lessons learned from six early adopters. Health Aff (Millwood) 2014;33(1):20–9.

24. Sage WM, Gallagher TH, Armstrong S, et al. How policy makers can smooth the way for communication-and-resolution programs. Health Aff (Millwood) 2014; 33(1):11–9.

25. McDonald TB, Helmchen LA, SMith KM, et al. Responding to patient safety incidents: the "seven pillars". Qual Saf Health Care 2010;19(6):e11.

26. Agency for Healthcare Research and Quality. Communication and Optimal Resolution (CANDOR) toolkit. 2017. Available at: http://www.ahrq.gov/professionals/quality-patient-safety/patient-safety-resources/resources/candor/introduction.html. Accessed February 28, 2019.

27. National Transportation Safety Board. The investigative process. Available at: https://www.ntsb.gov/investigations/process/Pages/default.aspx. Accessed February 28, 2019.

28. King S. Josie's story: a mother's crusade to make medical care safe. New York: Grove Press; 2009.

29. Graham P, Zerbi G, Norcross W, et al. Testing of a caregiver support team. Explore (NY) 2019;15(1):19–26.

30. Denham CR. TRUST: the 5 rights of the second victim. J Patient Saf 2007;3(2): 107–19.
31. Edrees H, Connors C, Paine L, et al. Implementing the RISE second victim support programme at the Johns Hopkins Hospital: a case study. BMJ Open 2016; 6(9):e011708. Available at: https://doi.org/10.1136/bmjopen-2016-011708. Accessed February 28, 2019.
32. Tamburri LM. Creating healthy work environments for second victims of adverse events. AACN Adv Crit Care 2017;28(4):366–74.

Implementation of the Confusion Assessment Method for Noncritically Ill Adult Patients

Katharine Outen, DNP, AGACNP-BC, AGCNS-BC[a],*,
Bimbola Fola Akintade, PhD, MBA, MHA, CCRN, ACNP-BC, NEA-BC[b,1]

KEYWORDS

- Delirium • Delirium screening • Confusion assessment method
- Delirium screening tool • Noncritically ill

KEY POINTS

- Experiencing delirium while hospitalized puts a patient at risk for increased morbidity and mortality. This also has negative financial effects.
- Routine screening is essential for early recognition of patients experiencing delirium.
- The Confusion Assessment Method is a reliable and widely used delirium screening tool that may help facilitate the necessary and effective management of delirium.
- The nurse-perceived usability of the Confusion Assessment Method for noncritically ill adult patients was above-average.

INTRODUCTION

For all hospitalized adults in the United States, the prevalence of delirium is estimated at 20%, with an incidence ranging from 18% to 64%.[1,2] It is also estimated that up to 80% of patients admitted to an intensive care unit (ICU) will experience delirium.[2] Delirium is a clinical syndrome characterized by acute onset fluctuations in mental status, accompanied by inattention, an altered level of consciousness, and impairment in cognition that is the direct physiologic consequence of a medical condition.[1] Several hospital interventions put a patient at risk for developing delirium, including mechanical ventilation, monitoring devices, medication interactions, use of physical restraints, urinary catheters, and interrupted sleep cycles.[3,4] Developing delirium increases a

Disclosure: The authors have nothing to disclose.
[a] University of Maryland Medical Center, Baltimore, MD 21201, USA; [b] University of Maryland School of Nursing, Baltimore, MD 21201, USA
[1] Present address: 655 West Lombard Street, Baltimore, MD 21201.
* Corresponding author. 22 South Greene Street, Baltimore, MD 21201.
E-mail address: kouten@umm.edu

Crit Care Nurs Clin N Am 31 (2019) 475–480
https://doi.org/10.1016/j.cnc.2019.07.002
0899-5885/19/© 2019 Elsevier Inc. All rights reserved.

patient's length of stay in an ICU, increases ventilator days, and increases overall hospital length of stay.[3,4] Untreated acute delirium can lead to seizures, coma, or even death; the inpatient mortality rate for individuals with delirium is estimated at 25% to 33%.[1,2] In the United States, the cost of delirium is estimated at $143 to $152 billion annually.[2,5]

Delirium is more than just an acute inpatient issue because the effects of delirium last long after the patient is discharged. A previous study found that patients who experience delirium during hospitalization have decreased cognition similar to those with mild Alzheimer disease and moderate traumatic brain injury up to 1 year after hospital discharge.[6] Experiencing delirium in the hospital has also been found to increase the risk of developing dementia in individuals aged 85 years and older and resulted in worsened dementia severity scores for individuals who previously had dementia.[7] Patients who experience delirium have a 5-fold increased risk of mortality following hospitalization and are more likely to need nursing home care after discharge.[1] Additionally, studies found that the longer a patient experiences delirium in the hospital, the higher the likelihood that they will have worsened cognition, executive functioning, ability to complete activities of daily living, and sensorimotor functioning after 1 year.[6,8,9]

Due to the high incidence of delirium in ICUs, patients are often routinely screened; however, it is inconsistently evaluated on inpatient hospital units. Due to the health and financial impacts, early recognition is key to preventing or reducing the effects of delirium. The aim of this quality improvement (QI) project was to implement and evaluate the nurse-perceived usability of the Confusion Assessment Method (CAM) delirium screening tool for noncritically ill adults on a medical intermediate care unit (MIMC).

METHODS

This QI project was conducted on a MIMC at a large academic hospital on the east coast of the United States. The project was designed to heighten the awareness of the need for delirium screening in the MIMC and, on completion, 80% of patients transferred to the MIMC from the medical ICU (MICU) would have a CAM screening completed.

Several delirium screening tools exist, but the CAM is the most widely used because it is a relatively simple, yet effective and reliable, tool; the CAM has a sensitivity of 95% and a specificity of 89%.[10–13]

A 13-week QI project was carried out on the 16-bed MIMC to evaluate the nurse-perceived usability of the CAM for noncritically ill adult patients. During the QI project implementation, bedside registered nurses (RNs) on the MIMC were asked to complete a CAM screening for each eligible patient they cared for each shift. The RN was then asked to complete the System Usability Scale (SUS) survey, a reliable and validated 10-item Likert-style questionnaire used to assess overall usability of a system intervention.[14] Each item on the SUS is ranked from 5 (strongly agree) to 1 (strongly disagree) and the scores are normalized to indicate overall usability.

The inclusion criteria for patients were all adult patients age 18 years and older who were transferred directly from the MICU to the MIMC. There were no exclusions of patients based on medical diagnosis. The patient sample size ($N = 183$) was determined by patient encounters; each 12-hour shift a patient was on the MIMC counted as 1 encounter. Inclusion criteria for the nurse survey sample to evaluate usability included the RNs who work on the MIMC and agreed to participate in the project. This sample size ($N = 181$) was determined by patient encounters and completion of a survey; each eligible patient an RN cared for per shift was counted as 1 survey, if the RN was willing to participate. The patient sample size (N = 183) and the RN survey sample size (N = 181) were not equal because for 2 eligible patient encounters in which a CAM screening tool was completed, the nurse did not complete a survey.

Volunteer unit champions were recruited for this QI project. The unit champions were trained on using the CAM delirium screening tool and, on completion, of the SUS survey by the project leader. The unit champions then assisted with educating the nursing staff on the MIMC regarding the QI project, as well as provide daily reminders to staff to participate in screening eligible patients.

Staff compliance with use of the CAM delirium screening tool was calculated by using the total number of completed CAMs divided by the total number of eligible patient encounters. The MIMC maintains a daily patient log of admissions and discharges that was used to evaluate the total number of patients that were eligible for delirium screening versus the total number of delirium screenings completed. Analysis of the SUS survey results included the total number completed and the overall percent usability. Additionally, the number of times a patient screened positive for delirium based on the CAM tools was noted.

RESULTS

There were a total of 329 eligible patient encounters during the implementation period. A total of 183 CAM screenings were completed, resulting in 55.6% compliance by the nursing staff. Of the 183 completed CAM screenings, 16 were positive, or suggestive of a diagnosis of delirium. This represents an 8.7% incidence of delirium for this patient population.

A total of 181 SUS surveys were completed by the nursing staff. Adjusted scores ranged from 35 to 100, with a mean rating of 77.94 ($SD \pm$ 12.21). According to the SUS tool instructions, a score greater than 68 indicates above-average usability. Of the 181 completed SUS surveys, 85.01% (n = 154) had adjusted scores higher than 68.

Each of the 10 questions of the SUS was also evaluated. For this QI project, the term system in the SUS survey referred to the CAM screening tool. For the first question, "I think I would like to use this system frequently," 67.9% (n = 123) selected "agree" or "strongly agree." For the second question, "I found this system unnecessarily complex," 89.5% (n = 162) selected "disagree" or "strongly disagree." For the third question, "I found this system easy to use," 92.8% (n = 168) selected "agree" or "strongly agree" (**Figs. 1** and **2**).

DISCUSSION

This QI project provides initial support regarding the nurse-perceived usability of the CAM screening tool for patients on a MIMC, with 85.01% (n = 154) of the 181 completed SUS surveys indicating above-average usability. Overall, RNs on the MIMC thought the CAM screening tool was useable within this patient population.

Previous studies estimated the prevalence of delirium at 20%, with incidence ranging from 18% to 64%.[1,2] This project found an incidence of 8.7%, which is markedly lower. However, this project only included patients transferred to the MIMC directly from the MICU, so it is possible the incidence rate would be higher if all patients on the MIMC were screened for delirium. RNs also noted that there were patients on the unit during the implementation period who did not meet inclusion criteria that would likely screen positive if they were included.

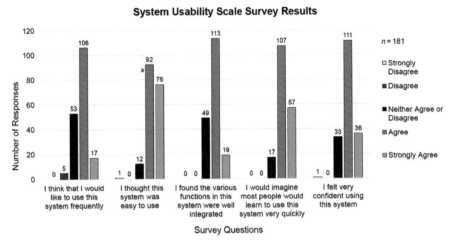

Fig. 1. RN responses on the SUS (questions 1–5).

Additionally, patients were only screened for delirium with the CAM tool for 9 weeks of the 13-week implementation period; the initial 4 weeks were dedicated to training of the unit champions and unit staff. The acuity of patient illness varies greatly on the MIMC, and it is possible that a longer data collection period would detect a higher incidence of delirium. Furthermore, for the duration of the implementation period, there were 2 patients on the unit who met inclusion requirements but were not experiencing delirium; these outliers may have lowered the incidence rate for the MIMC during the implementation period.

An unexpected finding of this project was that RN compliance with completing the CAM screening tool decreased after the midway point of implementation, despite reeducation of nursing staff. It was expected that compliance would increase as RNs became more familiar with the project and became more comfortable using the CAM screening tool. However, the unit had several weeks of understaffing during

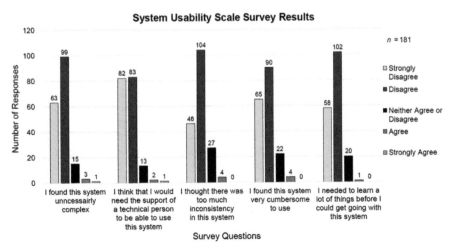

Fig. 2. RN responses on the SUS (questions 6–10).

the implementation period and, because project participation was voluntary, it is possible that staff elected not to participate in order to complete mandatory patient-related activities. Although staffing shortages are unavoidable, changing unit-based practice standards to include routine delirium screening on all patients would increase compliance. An electronic version of the CAM screening is already available in the electronic medical record (EMR) system used on the MIMC, so adoption into practice would be relatively simple and not create much change in the nursing workflow.

A strength noted with implementation of this project was the engagement of the charge RNs on the unit. The charge RNs noted eligible patients at daily change-of-shift huddles and reminded staff to participate by screening patients and completing the SUS survey. This engagement is crucial for sustainability and these individuals will likely be champions for changing unit-based practices to include delirium screening as part of routine nursing assessment in the future. This implementation also strengthened nurse collaboration within the unit and provided an opportunity for teaching and learning for all involved.

A limitation of this project was screening patients through the use of a paper CAM tool rather than within the EMR system. The paper form created an extra step in the nursing workflow, which may have decreased participation. Implementation of practice change can be met with more resistance when it changes workflows, so future studies to assess usability should incorporate delirium screening tools already available within EMR systems.

SUMMARY

Experiencing delirium negatively affects health outcomes for hospitalized adults. Early and ongoing identification of patients who may be experiencing delirium is crucial for delirium management and minimizing its long-term effects on cognition, executive functioning, and sensorimotor skills. Screening patients allows bedside RNs to implement preventive strategies, such as maintenance of sleep–wake cycles and promotion of mobility, in order to reduce the length of time a patient experiences delirium. The CAM was perceived as a useable screening tool for noncritically ill adult patients on a MIMC of a large, urban academic medical center on the east coast of the United States.

REFERENCES

1. American Psychiatric Association. Diagnostic and statistical manual of mental disorders. 5th eduion. Washington, DC: American Psychiatric Publishing; 2013.
2. Josephson SA, Miller BL. Confusion and delirium. In: Kasper DL, Fauci AS, Hauser SL, et al, editors. Harrison's principles of internal medicine. 19th edition. New York: McGraw-Hill; 2015. p. 166–70.
3. Anand A, MacLullich AMJ. Delirium in hospitalized older adults. Medicine 2017; 45(1):46–50.
4. Salluh JIF, Wang H, Schneider EB, et al. Outcome of delirium in critically ill patients: systematic review and meta-analysis. BMJ 2015;350:h2538.
5. Leslie DL, Inouye SK. The importance of delirium: economic and societal costs. J Am Geriatr Soc 2011;59(S2):S241–3.
6. Pandharipande PP, Girard TD, Jackson JC, et al. Long-term cognitive impairment after critical illness. N Engl J Med 2013;369:1306–16.

7. Davis DHJ, Terrera GM, Keage H, et al. Delirium is a strong risk-factor for dementia in the oldest-old: a population-based cohort study. Brain 2012;135(9):2809–16.
8. Brummel NE, Jackson JC, Pandharipande PP, et al. Delirium in the intensive care unit and subsequent long-term disability of survivors of mechanical ventilation. Crit Care Med 2014;42(2):369–77.
9. Vasilevskis EE, Han JH, Hughes CG, et al. Epidemiology and risk factors for delirium across hospital settings. Best Pract Res Clin Anaesthesiol 2012;26(3):277–87.
10. De J, Wand APF. Delirium screening: a systematic review of delirium screening tools in hospitalized patients. Gerontologist 2015;55(6):1079–99.
11. Holly C, Cantwell ER, Kamienski MC. Evidence-based practices for the identification, screening, and prevention of acute delirium in the hospitalized elderly: an overview of systematic reviews. Curr Transl Geriatr Exp Gerontol Rep 2013;2(1):7–15.
12. Inouye SK, Westendorp RGJ, Saczynski JS. Delirium in elderly people. Lancet 2014;383(9920):911–22.
13. Kalish VB, Gillham JE, Unwin BK. Delirium in older persons: evaluation and management. Am Fam Physician 2014;90(3):150–8.
14. Bangor A, Kortum PT, Miller JT. An empirical evaluation of the system usability scale. Int J Hum Comput Interact 2008;24(6):574–94.

Assessing Nursing and Pediatric Resident Understanding of Delirium in the Pediatric Intensive Care Unit

Molly E. McGetrick, MD[a,b,]*, Caitlin Lach, BSN, RN[c,d],
Jodi E. Mullen, RN-BC[c], Jennifer C. Munoz-Pareja, MD[e]

KEYWORDS

- Pediatrics • Delirium • Critical care • Intensive care • Benzodiazepines • Education
- Nursing

KEY POINTS

- Delirium is a widespread illness state in the pediatric intensive care unit, although it often goes unrecognized by providers.
- The diagnosis of delirium in children is often difficult because of features of acute illness, medications used, varied developmental stages among patients, and lack of universally used screening practices.
- Both pediatric intensive care nurses and pediatric residents have variable experience in recognizing and treating delirium, highlighting an important educational opportunity.
- Education on the risk factors for delirium and appropriate management should improve provider comfort, while improving patient experiences and outcomes in the intensive care unit.

INTRODUCTION

Among patients in the pediatric intensive care unit (ICU), delirium is common and is associated with significant morbidity. Small studies have shown the incidence in the pediatric ICU often exceeds 30%.[1–3] Delirium has been shown to incur higher hospital costs, even when controlled for primary diagnosis and length of stay, and may also have long-term effects on the health of individuals who experience

Disclosure Statement: The authors have nothing to disclose.
[a] Division of Pediatrics, University of Florida, Gainesville, FL, USA; [b] Division of Pediatric Critical Care, University of Texas Southwestern, Dallas, TX, USA; [c] University of Florida, Shands Children's Hospital, 1600 Southwest Archer Road, Gainesville, FL 32608, USA; [d] College of Nursing, University of Florida, Gainesville, FL, USA; [e] Division of Pediatric Critical Care, Department of Pediatrics, University of Florida, 1600 Southwest Archer Road, Gainesville, FL 32608, USA
* Corresponding author. 1935 Medical District Drive, Dallas, TX 75235.
E-mail address: Molly.mcgetrick@UTsouthwestern.edu

Crit Care Nurs Clin N Am 31 (2019) 481–488
https://doi.org/10.1016/j.cnc.2019.07.003
0899-5885/19/© 2019 Elsevier Inc. All rights reserved.

the disease state.[1,4,5] However, even though delirium is an expensive and injurious problem, studies have shown that there are drastic variations in education and screening practices in pediatric ICUs.[1,5–8] Furthermore, it has been shown that there are measurable knowledge gaps among health care providers in the pediatric ICU.[6,7] Targeted educational initiatives can improve baseline knowledge and provider comfort in caring for the delirious pediatric patient. When successful, these interventions will likely lead to better care and better long-term outcomes for patients who receive care in the ICU.[6,7]

The primary aim of this survey-based study was to assess the delirium knowledge base of pediatric residents and ICU nurses at a medium-sized academic pediatric hospital. Secondarily, the authors sought to assess provider comfort in identifying delirium as well as presumed frequency of interactions with delirious patients.

MATERIALS AND METHODS

This survey-based study was conducted between March and April 2017. Survey participants were pediatric residents in a medium-sized academic residency program, and nursing staff from a 24-bed pediatric ICU and a 22-bed pediatric cardiac ICU in the respective teaching hospital. A 20-question survey was prepared to assess knowledge of tools and diagnostic criteria for delirium, risk factors, presumed incidence of delirium, and overall staff comfort with the diagnosis and management of delirium. The first 17 questions were adopted from the survey used in a similar study by Flaigle and colleagues,[6] who administered their survey to the pediatric ICU nursing staff at a large academic institution. Three additional questions were added that assessed provider comfort with delirium identification, presumed frequency of interactions with delirious patients, and multiple-choice responses to assess what supplemental measures can be used for delirium prevention and management.

Deidentified surveys were distributed to the nursing staff during their working shift, and participation was voluntary. Individuals provided verbal consent to participate. Similarly, 53 pediatric residents at this same institution were asked to participate in the same survey, which was posted on the online polling Web site, Survey Monkey (http://www.surveymonkey.com). All responses were anonymous and not tracked to individual residents.

Data were summarized as the percentage of individuals who received correct answers on questions 1 to 17 (**Table 1**). Responses to questions 18 to 20 were analyzed separately (**Tables 2** and **3**). The results obtained from this study were used to create target educational materials for the nursing staff in both the pediatric ICU and the pediatric cardiac ICU. These materials include paper handouts and online presentations, which became part of the required continuing education for the nursing staff. For pediatric residents, informal introductions to delirium screening and management are provided during their required rotation through the ICU.

RESULTS

The individuals who completed the survey included 73 nurses who work primarily in the pediatric ICU or pediatric cardiac ICU, and 32 general pediatric residents. Among the nursing staff and pediatric resident physicians, the survey response rate was 46.2% (73/158) and 60.3% (32/53), respectively. Pediatric residents were further subdivided based on their year in training: 25.8% of participants were in postgraduate year 1 (PGY-1), 45.16% were in PGY-2, and 29.03% were in PGY-3.

Table 1
Results of delirium survey

	Pediatric Residents (%)	Nurses (%)	Total (%)
1. Fluctuation between orientation and disorientation is not typical of delirium. (False)	29 (90.6)	67 (91.7)	96 (91.4)
2. Poor nutrition increases the risk of delirium. (True)	32 (100)	70 (95.8)	102 (97.1)
3. The GCS score is the best way to diagnose delirium in critically ill children. (False)	30 (93.7)	67 (91.7)	97 (92.3)
4. Hearing or vision impairment increases the risk of delirium. (True)	31 (96.9)	68 (93.1)	99 (94.3)
5. Delirium in children always manifests as a hyperactive, confused state. (False)	32 (100)	71 (97.2)	103 (98.1)
6. Benzodiazepines can be helpful in the treatment of delirium. (False)	23 (71.9)	34 (46.6)	57 (54.3)
7. Behavioral changes in the course of the day are typical of delirium. (True)	32 (100)	68 (93.1)	100 (95.2)
8. Patients with delirium will often experience perceptual disturbances. (True)	30 (93.7)	71 (97.2)	101 (96.2)
9. Altered sleep/wake cycle may be a symptom of delirium. (True)	32 (100)	73 (100)	105 (100)
10. Symptoms of depression may mimic delirium. (True)	31 (96.9)	70 (95.8)	101 (96.2)
11. The greater number of medications, the greater their risk of delirium. (True)	31 (96.9)	71 (97.2)	102 (97.1)
12. Delirium usually lasts several hours. (False)	16 (50)	38 (52.0)	54 (51.4)
13. A urinary catheter in situ reduces the risk of delirium. (False)	28 (87.5)	71 (97.2)	99 (94.3)
14. Gender has no effect on the development of delirium. (False)	23 (71.9)	24 (32.8)	47 (44.8)
15. Dehydration can be a risk factor for delirium. (True)	31 (96.9)	73 (100)	104 (99.0)
16. Children generally do not remember being delirious. (False)	9 (28.1)	18 (24.6)	27 (25.7)
17. A family history of dementia predisposes a patient to delirium. (False)	23 (71.9)	41 (56.6)	64 (61.0)

Collectively, most participants correctly identified that contributing factors for delirium include poor nutritional status (97.1%; n = 102), sensory impairment (94.3%; n = 99), and polypharmacy (97.1%, n = 102). Of the 17 discrete questions, there were 2 for which 100% of respondents answered correctly: altered sleep-wake cycle may be a symptom of delirium (true) and dehydration may be a risk factor for delirium (true). The maximum and minimum scores for both the nursing and the

Table 2
Provider responses to "how comfortable do you feel that you would be able to identify a patient with delirium?"

	Very Comfortable, %	Somewhat Comfortable, %	Not Very Comfortable, %	Extremely Uncomfortable, %
Residents	0 (0)	53.1 (17)	46.9 (15)	0 (0)
Nurses	1.4 (1)	65.7 (48)	31.5 (23)	1.4 (1)

Table 3
Provider responses to "how often do you think you observe a patient with delirium?"

	More than Once a Week, %	About Once a Week, %	Less than Once a Week but More than Once a Month, %	Once a Month or Fewer, %	I Have Never Seen a Patient with Delirium, %
Residents	0 (0)	9.4 (3)	12.5 (4)	62.5 (20)	15.6 (5)
Nurses	4.1 (3)	16.4 (12)	30.1 (22)	46.6 (34)	2.7 (2)

resident cohorts were 94% (16/17 correct) and 65% (11/17 correct), respectively. Of the pediatric residents surveyed, the average score was 85%, and the nursing staff averaged at 79.5% on these 17 questions. Overall, there were 5 questions (see questions 6, 12, 14, 16 and 17 in **Table 1**) for which greater than 25% of participants from both groups answered incorrectly.

For most of the questions, there were similar percentages of correct and incorrect responses between the resident and nursing groups. However, the largest discrepancies between the 2 groups were the responses to the statements "benzodiazepines can be helpful in the treatment of delirium," "gender has no effect on the development of delirium," and "a family history of dementia predisposes a patient to delirium." For these survey questions, a larger proportion of residents answered correctly, with a difference in correct answers between resident and nursing staff of 25.3%, 39.1%, and 15.3%, respectively. Nursing staff more frequently identified that urinary catheters and dehydration are risk factors for delirium and that delirium is a state that usually does not last several hours.

When comparing the 2 groups of providers surveyed, the ICU nursing staff reported a greater degree of comfort in identifying a delirious patient, with 67.1% answering that they were either very comfortable or somewhat comfortable with this task. By comparison, only 53% of residents responded similarly. Within the authors' cohort, 46% of pediatric residents and 32.5% of nurses listed that they were either not very comfortable or extremely uncomfortable with their own abilities to identify a patient with delirium.

The final question of this survey was a multiple response item, which assessed perceived benefit of supplemental interventions for reducing and managing delirium (**Fig. 1**). Responses varied, but most individuals reported that physical therapy, music, and measures to reduce excessive sensory stimuli, such as eye masks and earplugs, were beneficial. For all but one of the choices in this question, a greater proportion of nursing staff answered correctly, although more residents reported correctly that physical therapy was a beneficial intervention for the management of delirium. A small, but significant, number of respondents incorrectly identified sedation, benzodiazepines, and frequent daytime napping as beneficial measures.

DISCUSSION

Delirium is defined as a syndrome of acute cerebral dysfunction with alterations in baseline mental status, attention, and cognition.[8] Often, this is brought about by the conditions that bring a child into the ICU, but can be further provoked by necessary medical therapies, alterations in sleep-wake cycles during care, and baseline developmental delays or psychiatric disorders. Although delirium affects up to 30% of children hospitalized in ICUs, studies have shown that the condition remains underdiagnosed in the pediatric population.[1,3–6,8] Although there are many potentially contributive interventions that cannot be completely eliminated, that is, withholding of necessary

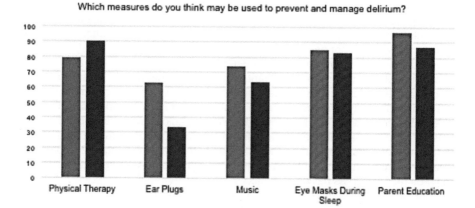

Fig. 1. Nursing and resident perception of the utility of certain interventions for the management and prevention of delirium. Each bar quantifies the percentages of respondents from each group who thought that the above interventions were beneficial.

sedation or decreasing frequency of hands-on activities during critical periods of illness, improved education for individuals caring for children in this setting can help providers gain a better understanding of the disease process. Likewise, informed providers are more likely to be proactive and advocate for the best care for their patients. In order to deliver maximal benefit with educational initiatives, knowledge gaps need to be identified in all provider levels.

Before the creation of this study, Flaigle and colleagues[6] demonstrated that, at a large academic institution, there were significant knowledge gaps regarding the diagnosis and management of delirium. Among their findings, they stated that 38% of survey respondents reported that benzodiazepines were beneficial for delirium treatment; 11% thought that the Glasgow Coma Scale (GCS) is an appropriate delirium screening method, and 62% responded that they did not think children remembered being delirious. During the conception of the follow-up study, the authors assumed that they would achieve similar results at their institution. Based on the survey responses obtained, the authors indeed found that a significant knowledge gaps exist in their institution among pediatric intensive care nurses as well as pediatric residents who rotate through the pediatric ICU during their training. Perhaps the most striking finding was that 46% of participants pooled thought that benzodiazepines could be beneficial in the treatment of delirium, despite the fact that these medications have been associated with higher incidences of delirium, prolonged delirium course, and lower rates of ICU discharge.[9] This, along with other survey responses, did indeed confirm the authors' suspicion that a similar pattern was present from the former study.

The lack of provider knowledge in the authors' institution and other similar institutions is likely multifactorial. Although delirium is a topic that is covered in baseline medical and nursing education, training is often limited, and in many cases, the subject is taught in the context of adult patients. This pattern of teaching may lead to a baseline assumption that delirium is a disease of old age. In most pediatric ICUs, few, if any, educational resources about delirium are provided to nursing providers as part of orientation and continued education. In the absence of routine screening for delirium, which occurs in less than 30% of pediatric ICUs, the lack of familiarity with formal screening tools contributes to a reduced understanding of cardinal features and behaviors of a delirious patient.[8] With that, the behaviors displayed by a delirious patient, such as decreased activity, agitation, and decreased awareness of surroundings, may be assumed by providers to be a usual manifestation of primary illness, and therefore, not addressed in an appropriate manner.

Beyond the gaps in provider training, there are features unique to the pediatric critical care population that makes the identification of delirium difficult. These features include various developmental stages, high rates of children with cognitive delays, state of high disability, and the presence or absence of home caregivers. With all of these factors involved, it can be difficult to expect medical and nursing providers to assess a delirious patient based on observation alone, although recognition of the risk factors is the first step. Among the children in the ICU, those aged 2 to 5 years, those requiring mechanical ventilation, and those with baseline developmental delays should be recognized as having high risk.[1,2,4,5,8]

Before the initiation of this study, there was no protocol or instrument in place at the authors' institution for identifying pediatric patients experiencing delirium. Therefore, it is not surprising that in the authors' study, 47% of the participants said they were not very comfortable or extremely uncomfortable with the task identifying a child experiencing delirium. Use of standardized tools, including the Cornell Assessment of Pediatric Delirium (CAP-D), the Pediatric Confusion Assessment Method–Intensive Care Unit, and the Pediatric Anesthesia Emergence Delirium Scale, help to remove some of the provider anxiety with making a diagnosis based on observation alone and regiment the process of screening pediatric patients for delirium.[4,6–8] Since conducting this assessment in the authors' pediatric ICUs, they have implemented a formal screening protocol for delirium using the CAP-D and increased the amount of formal nurse and resident education. It is expected that these interventions will increase provider awareness of delirium and allow them to identify this condition on a more consistent basis. Follow-up assessments are pending at this time.

Aside from the knowledge of assessment of delirium, providers also play a role in promoting the use of supplemental measures to prevent and mitigate delirium symptoms in patients. The first step in delirium prevention involves efforts to maintain a level of sedation whereby the patient is calm, yet alert when at all possible. Medical providers should work closely with the nursing staff to ensure that the medication regimen is optimized to achieve this goal, while avoiding deliriogenic medications when possible. Nursing and support staff can further advocate for the patient by encouraging environmental modifications that promote a healthy sleep-wake cycle (providing ear plugs, face mask, and calming music), encouraging early physical therapy when possible, and educating parents on the signs and symptoms of delirium, while encouraging their participation in the patient's care.[2,8] Although literature demonstrates that these supplemental measures can be beneficial, the results of the authors' study showed that less than 80% of providers surveyed thought that physical therapy, music, and earplugs were useful in delirium management. Not surprisingly, the nursing staff surveyed scored generally higher in these areas, which may be reflective of their observation of the utility of these measures for this, and other similar disease states (see **Fig. 1**).[6–8]

Overall, there remains a significant need to educate institutions' pediatric intensive care nurses and pediatric residents about delirium and its management. This educational goal aligns with the goals of other children's hospitals, which are now recognizing delirium as a significant problem affecting pediatric patients and are taking steps to prevent and treat the condition.[10,11] It is evident that at the authors' institution, room for growth exists in combating delirium in children hospitalized in the ICUs. The approach to education must be multifactorial and should include interprofessional strategies to incorporate all members of the health care team. These interventions may include, but are not limited to, standard practice guidelines, multiprofessional rounds, and empowering team members invested in promoting delirium education to all providers in the ICU.[8] In addition, pediatric residents should be encouraged to use evidence-based practices and advocate for sedation protocols that minimize the use of benzodiazepines when possible. With these measures, members of pediatric ICUs can support a movement toward improved delirium prevention as well as discover and use more effective treatment modalities.

Limitations to this study include a lack of full participation by pediatric ICU nurses and pediatric residents. As such, the results of this study may not be generalizable to all pediatric intensive care nurses and pediatric residents in the authors' institution and in others. Although the authors attempted to capture a large sample of the nursing staff, there may have been some innate selection bias and may not represent the entirety of the spectrum from new nursing staff, to those with the most experience. Likewise, the resident provider arm may have been biased because those who had more interest or were more knowledgeable in the area of delirium may have been more likely to complete the voluntary survey. In addition, data from this study were taken at 1 time point, with no data on health care provider knowledge about delirium being collected after additional education is complete. Despite the fact that the authors' results partially mirrored the survey study by Flaigle and colleagues,[6] it may not be generalizable to all institutions, especially those who are already actively screening for delirium on a routine basis.

SUMMARY

A significant factor in the underrecognition of delirium is a lack of provider knowledge about the condition, including its prevention, assessment, and treatment. The authors' study demonstrates that this knowledge gap exists in their institution among both pediatric intensive care nurses and pediatric residents. The authors suspect that this has negative implications on patient care, because delirium in children admitted in the authors' institution's pediatric ICUs is likely underdiagnosed and undertreated. The authors' results highlight a need for improved delirium education across all levels of training to improve recognition, treatment, and provider comfort in caring for the delirious pediatric patient. Although delirium has recently gained wide recognition in the pediatric intensive care community, the authors suspect that other institutions may still benefit from assessing the knowledge of their providers, in order to implement targeted educational initiatives.

REFERENCES

1. Traube C, Silver G, Kearney J, et al. Cornell assessment of pediatric delirium: a valid, rapid, observational tool for screening delirium in the PICU. Crit Care Med 2014;42(3):656–63.
2. Schieveld JNM, Leroy PLJM, Van OS J, et al. Pediatric delirium in critical care illness: phenomenology, clinical correlates and treatment response in the pediatric intensive care unit. Intensive Care Med 2007;33:1022–1040l.
3. Hatherhill S, Flisher AJ. Delirium in children and adolescents: a systematic review of the literature. J Psychosom Res 2010;68:337–44.
4. Silver G, Kearney J, Traube C, et al. Delirium screening anchored in child development: the Cornell Assessment of Pediatric Delirium. Palliat Support Care 2015;13(4):1005–11.
5. Traube C, Mauer EA, Gerber LM, et al. Cost associated with pediatric delirium in the intensive care unit. Crit Care Med 2016;44(12):e1175–9.

6. Flaigle MC, Ascenzi J, Kudchakar SR. Identifying barriers to delirium screening and prevention in the pediatric ICU: evaluation of PICU staff knowledge. J Pediatr Nurs 2016;31:81–4.
7. Simone S, Edwards S, Lardieri A, et al. Implementation of an ICU bundle: an interprofessional quality improvement project to enhance management and monitor delirium prevalence in a single PICU. Pediatr Crit Care Med 2017;18(6):531–40.
8. Bettencourt A, Mullen J. Delirium in children: identification, prevention, and management. Crit Care Nurse 2017;37(3):e9–18.
9. Smith HAB, Gangopadhyay M, Goben CM, et al. Delirium and benzodiazepines associated with prolonged ICU stay in critically ill infants and young children. Crit Care Med 2017;45(9):1427–35.
10. Owens T, Tapley C. Pediatric mobility: the development of standard assessments and interventions for pediatric patients for safe patient handling and mobility. Crit Care Nurs Q 2018;41(3):314–22.
11. Wolfe H, Mack A, Warrington S, et al. PICU/PCU delirium pathway. Children's Hospital of Philadelphia. 2017. Available at: https://www.chop.edu/clinical-pathway/picu-pcu-delirium-clinical-pathway. Accessed January 15, 2019.

Sarcopenia and Psychosocial Variables in Patients in Intensive Care Units

The Role of Nutrition and Rehabilitation in Prevention and Treatment

Sareen Gropper, PhD-Nutrition, RDN, LDN[a], Dennis Hunt, EdD, CSCS[b],
Deborah W. Chapa, PhD, ACNP-BC, ACHPN[c],*

KEYWORDS

- Enteral nutrition • Early mobilization • Cognitive decline • Sarcopenia

KEY POINTS

- Protein and mobility prevent sarcopenia and cognitive decline in intensive care unit patients.
- Two others Adequate protein intake may be vital to prevent sarcopenia in critically ill patients.
- Increased mobility is an important part of sarcopenia prevention in critically ill patients.

Critical illness refers generally to medical conditions necessitating treatment in the surgical intensive care unit (ICU) or medical ICU. These conditions often include sepsis, major burns and trauma, ischemia, hemorrhage, severe tissue injuries such as pancreatitis, and organ failure along with some postsurgical states. With advances in practice, ICU-associated mortality rates have declined over the years, and more ICU patients are surviving and being discharged. Coupled with these improvements in survival, however, are increases in ICU-acquired conditions affecting the physical function, cognitive function, and quality of life of the survivors. This article reviews (1) the response to critical illness with a focus on muscle, (2) ICU outcomes with a focus on muscle, (3) the added

Disclosure Statement: The authors have nothing to disclose.
[a] Christine E. Lynn College of Nursing, Florida Atlantic University, Building 84, Office 322, 777 Glades Road, Boca Raton, FL 33431, USA; [b] Florida Gulf Coast University, 10501 FGCU Boulevard South, Fort Myers, FL 33965, USA; [c] Lee Health, 8925 Colonial Center Drive, Building A, Suite 1000, Fort Myers, FL 33905, USA
* Corresponding author.
E-mail address: deborah.chapa@leehealth.org

Crit Care Nurs Clin N Am 31 (2019) 489–499
https://doi.org/10.1016/j.cnc.2019.07.004
0899-5885/19/© 2019 Elsevier Inc. All rights reserved.

impact of older age with a focus on muscle, (4) approaches to identifying those at nutritional risk, (5) dietary protein and critical illness, and (6) implications for practice.

RESPONSE TO CRITICAL ILLNESS WITH A FOCUS ON MUSCLE

Critical illness has a profound impact on the body's tissues. Although this impact varies in degree depending on the nature and extent of the illness or injury, skeletal muscle mass is affected dramatically and quickly on onset of the illness/injury. In healthy individuals, skeletal muscle enables physical function, and the ingestion of protein-rich foods provides the body with the amino acids that are needed to maintain skeletal muscle mass, strength, and function. In those patients with critical illness, however, this physical functional role of skeletal muscle is overshadowed by its need to serve as a protein pool or reservoir that can be readily catabolized to supply the body's other tissues with amino acids. Muscle's role as a pool/reservoir is vital because the body does not store or have extra/reserve proteins (amino acids) available in times of heightened needs.

The body's initial reactions to critical illness occur in response to the neuroendocrine and immune systems and involve the release of several catabolic hormones, including glucagon, epinephrine, and cortisol, as well as several proinflammatory cytokines, such as interleukin (IL)-1 and IL-6, interferons, and tumor necrosis factor α. The hormonal response triggers the catabolism of glycogen stores, adipose tissue, and muscle to provide nutrient substrates for use by the brain, heart, and other vital organs. This proinflammatory/catabolic environment in critical illness also contributes to metabolic derangements, such as insulin resistance, hyperglycemia, and impaired fatty acid oxidation. Moreover, it facilitates the chronic assault on the body's skeletal muscle mass, reducing the synthesis and promoting the degradation of muscle proteins. The cytokine tumor necrosis factor α, for example, and myostatin (an inhibitory growth factor) binds to separate receptors on muscle cells to trigger a series of reactions that ultimately increase the activity of the ubiquitin proteasomal pathway. This pathway is responsible for most protein degradation within muscle. Cortisol and glucagon also trigger protein degradation via the up-regulation of lysosomal autophagy in many nonmuscle tissues.

The amount of skeletal muscle mass that is catabolized in periods of critical illness can be quite large and typically occurs to the greatest extent within the first 10 days.[1–4] Losses of 1.62 kg (15.5%) of total body protein (with 1.09 kg [67%] of the total from skeletal muscle) were found over a period of 21 days in 10 patients admitted to the ICU with trauma.[1] Reductions of 10.3% in the cross-sectional area of the rectus femoris (part of the quadriceps complex) and 17.5% decreases in muscle fibers have been reported in critically ill patients (most of whom had sepsis) on day 7 of hospitalization in the ICU.[2] In another group of 20 patients admitted to the ICU with sepsis and trauma, total body protein losses averaged 13.1% and 14.6%, respectively, at the end of a 21-day period.[4]

These losses of skeletal muscle observed in adults (especially older adults) with critical illness are much higher than the losses that occur with bed rest alone (ie, nonpathologic muscle disuse). For example, when compared with values prior to 20 days of bed rest, 12 healthy older adults (mean 67 years) lost 1500 g of lean mass, of which 950 g (63%) come from muscle in the lower extremities.[5] Losses in muscle strength and significant decreases in muscle protein synthesis were also reported despite a protein intake of 0.8 g/kg body weight, consistent with the recommended dietary allowance.[5] The loss of muscle mass observed in these older adults is substantially greater than the 400 g of lean leg mass loss that was reported in 6 healthy younger adults who underwent 28 days of bed rest.[6]

The draining of the muscle protein pool/reservoir in critical illness provides for the release of amino acids, which are then directed to the liver, bone marrow, spleen, and lymph nodes, among other organs/tissues for use in the synthesis of glucose and life-sustaining proteins (eg, acute-phase proteins, immunologic proteins, and proteins involved in wound repair and healing). The liver, for example, increases production of (positive) acute-phase proteins, such as C-reactive protein, fibrinogen, plasminogen activator inhibitor, haptoglobin, and amyloid A, among others, and reduces its synthesis of less critical proteins like albumin and prealbumin. This proinflammatory phase of critical illness (especially common in those with severe trauma, burns, and sepsis) is referred to as systemic inflammatory response syndrome (SIRS) and leads to the development of multiple organ failure in many patients. The return of immune system homeostasis enables patient recovery from SIRS; however, some patients exhibit persistent or ongoing inflammation and suppression of adaptive immunity. This situation increases the risk of persistent inflammation, immunosuppression, and catabolism syndrome (PICS). PICS is a chronic critical illness (>2 weeks in duration) characterized by organ dysfunction, immunosuppression (lymphopenia), low-grade inflammation (neutrophilia), an ongoing acute-phase protein response (high C-reactive protein and hypoalbuminemia), and prolonged body protein catabolism.[7] Compensatory anti-inflammatory response syndrome, a syndrome in which the release of anti-inflammatory mediators overcompensates for the systemic inflammatory response, also may occur in critically ill patients and can result in immunosuppression (increasing susceptibility to further infection) and impaired recovery.

The muscle loss observed in critically ill ICU patients, whether occurring in response to the (previously discussed) increased concentrations of catabolic hormone and cytokines, inflammation, and muscle disuse (bedrest) and/or in combination with reductions in blood flow, use of neuromuscular blockers or corticosteroids, and inadequate protein intake, worsens patient outcomes. Survivors of the ICU can face months to years of physical rehabilitation.

INTENSIVE CARE UNIT OUTCOMES WITH A FOCUS ON MUSCLE

The changes in the body's use of amino acids in critical illness help facilitate recovery but simultaneously result in skeletal muscle mass loss and weakness. The development of PICS prolongs the catabolic effects on muscle. PICS also is associated with reductions in functional status, poor wound healing, recurrent nosocomial infections, and increased risk of pressure ulcers.[7]

ICU-acquired weakness (ICUAW) is another outcome seen in ICU survivors. The condition is characterized by myopathy and/or polyneuropathy especially affecting the lower limbs. The polyneuropathy is characterized by primary axonal degeneration, with effects on motor neurons to a greater extent than sensory neurons. Muscles exhibit a loss of thick muscle fibers (myosin proteins) and diminished excitability with direct stimulation, resulting in loss of muscle mass, strength, and function.[8] The causes and pathophysiology of ICUAW are multifactorial. The use of medications, especially glucocorticoids and neuromuscular blocking agent, prolonged immobilization, and joint contractures as well as the metabolic effects associated with hyperglycemia, systemic inflammation, and oxidative stress are thought to contribute to ICUAW.[8,9] ICUAW results in functional disability, including reduced abilities to perform activities of daily living and instrumental activities of daily living, and may persist after discharge from the ICU.[10] Greater trajectories of cognitive impairments also have been found 1 year post–ICU stay in individuals treated for severe sepsis versus those hospitalized for noncritical illness.[11] Individuals with PICS or ICUAW, among other post-ICU conditions, usually are discharged to long-term care facilities, with poor outcomes.[7] Even with rehabilitation, most, especially older, adults do not attain pre-ICU functional status.[8]

THE ADDED IMPACT OF OLDER AGE WITH A FOCUS ON MUSCLE

Older versus younger patients admitted to the ICU experience greater obstacles given they are more likely to have been admitted with preexisting conditions that have affected muscle. One such condition is sarcopenia, which typically occurs with aging and affects up to 70% of older adults.[12,13] Sarcopenia is characterized by reductions in muscle mass, strength, and/or function. The changes in muscle include losses of type II fast-twitch muscle fibers and of motor neurons. These losses occur to a greater extent in lower versus upper limb muscle groups and are substantial.[14,15] Lean muscle mass in young adults, for example, represents close to 50% of body mass; in contrast, in adults 75 years to 80 years of age, lean mass accounts for only approximately 25% of body mass.[14,15] Thus, older adults with preexisting sarcopenia who are admitted to the ICU face even more challenges given the damaging effects of critical illness on an already reduced muscle mass.

Losses of muscle mass and strength, whether primary or secondary to critical illness, are associated with multiple adverse consequences during the postrecovery period from critical illness. Sarcopenia increases the risk of falls, fractures, and frailty and is associated with increased risk for infections, prolonged length of hospital stay, increased hospital costs, a greater likelihood of rehospitalization, and increased mortality.[16] Recent studies also show that declines in muscle strength and physical function have a negative impact on brain health, including cognition and development of dementia.[17,18]

Another preexisting condition common among older adults and characterized by reductions in muscle mass is malnutrition. Up to 50% (and perhaps more) of patients are admitted to the hospital with preexisting malnutrition, secondary to either inadequate nutrient/protein intake and/or chronic illness.[19–21] Once hospitalized, the malnutrition can worsen in those who were already malnourished or can develop secondary to insufficient protein and nutrient intakes needed because of acute medical conditions (disease or injury) or inflammation.[22] Protein malnutrition further reduces muscle mass, impairs immune system function, increases the likelihood of infection, reduces wound healing, increases the risk of pressure ulcers, increases complication rates, increases length of hospital stay, and increases morbidity and mortality.[20]

IDENTIFICATION OF THOSE AT NUTRITIONAL RISK

The risk of mortality as well as of developing complications, such as prolonged mechanical ventilation/weaning failure, immunosuppression, infections, longer length of stay, and muscle weakness, is higher among ICU patients who are identified as at nutritional risk or at high risk.[23–25] Early identification of these at-risk or high-risk ICU patients coupled with the provision of adequate nutrition support can help improve patient outcomes.[24,26] Although prospective randomized controlled studies are needed, the Nutrition Risk in Critical Care (NUTRIC) and the modified NUTRIC (mNUTRIC) represent validated screening options to identify critically ill patients who are at nutritional risk and who would benefit most from higher nutrient intakes.[27–29] NUTRIC considers a patient's age, Acute Physiology and Chronic Health

Evaluation II score, sequential organ failure assessment score, number of comorbidities, time in the hospital prior to the ICU admission, and blood IL-6 concentrations.[30] The modified version does not include IL-6 concentrations. High scores, 6 to 10 on the NUTRIC and 5 to 9 on the mNUTRIC, have been associated with worse clinical outcomes.[29] Screening in those at risk should be followed by nutritional assessment, for example, using the subjective global assessment tool and other pertinent medical information vital for consideration in providing nutritional support.[28] The use of ultrasonography at the bedside in the ICU setting and computed tomography scans has provided a means for the identification of critically ill patients at highest risk for developing ICUAW.[3,31] Muscle quantity and quality, for example, can be detected using ultrasonography and have been associated with functional and clinical outcomes.[31]

DIETARY PROTEIN AND CRITICAL ILLNESS

Sufficient quantities and the correct proportions of amino acids along with energy must be present in body cells for the synthesis of proteins. Although the exact or optimal amount of dietary protein that is needed for critically ill patients has not been clearly established, recommendations for critically ill patients (in the absence of liver and renal failure) arising from the International Protein Summit clearly and consistently suggest the provision of protein of at least 1.2 g/kg body weight to 2.0 g/kg body weight, with such intakes achieved by the fourth day of ICU admission if feasible.[19,26,32–34] Given recommendations for protein intake for geriatric patients with acute and chronic diseases who are not critically ill range from 1.2 g/kg body weight to 1.5 g/kg body weight, it is likely that older critically ill patients may need initial intakes of at least 1.5 g/kg body weight per day.[35,36]

Higher initial protein intakes, starting, for example, with at least 1.5 g/kg body weight have been suggested for those with PICS and preexisting conditions such as sarcopenia.[7,35] Even higher protein intakes, at 2.0 g/kg body weight to 2.5 g/kg body weight, are thought to be needed for patients with severe sepsis, extensive burns, and multiple trauma.[32] Because overestimation of protein needs in critically ill patients who are obese can occur with the use of the weight-based calculation, the substitution of ideal body weight in place of actual body weight may be needed. Initial protein recommendations for critically ill patients with a body mass index (BMI) of 30 kg/m^2 to 39.9 kg/m^2 are 2.0 g/kg ideal body weight and for those with a BMI greater than or equal to 40 kg/m^2 are 2.5 g/kg body weight.[32] Although additional studies to more precisely identify protein recommendations are still needed, more practical solutions are needed to ensure that the patients receive sufficient nutrition to meet the nutrient prescriptions. A comparison of prescribed protein recommendations versus current practice reflected a bleak picture of iatrogenic underfeeding, with evaluations of current feeding practices to critically ill patients in hospitals worldwide showing significant inadequacies.[37–42] In an investigation of 187 ICUs across the globe, which included approximately 4000 patients, prescriptions for protein intake averaged 1.3 g/kg body weight per day; however, patients received on average only approximately 55% (range 15% to 101%) of the prescribed protein.[29] Moreover, only approximately 16% of the patients received more than 80% of prescribed energy needs,[29] suggesting improvements are needed in the delivery of nutrition to critically ill patients and that the actual delivery (vs the prescription) of nutrition support must be monitored.[29]

The provision of higher dietary protein to critically ill patients has been shown to provide benefits in several studies. For example, higher protein (1.2 g/kg body weight) and energy (21 kcal/kg body weight) intakes versus standard of care (0.75 g/kg and 18 kcal/kg) in critically ill patients resulted in significantly better attenuation of quadriceps muscle layer thickness and significantly lower prevalence of malnutrition at discharge from the ICU.[33]

Higher protein intakes, at 1.1 g/kg body weight versus 0.9 g/kg body weight over a 1-week period, resulted in statistically significantly greater forearm muscle thickness and less fatigue, and, although not statistically significant, improvements in grip strength in a double-blind randomized controlled trial involving 119 critically ill patients in the ICU.[34] A multicenter, multinational study reported that a higher protein intake was associated with reduced infectious complications, length of stay in the ICU, and mortality in high-risk, critically ill patients.[42,43] Studies in survivors of the ICU have also shown benefits, including decreased mortality from greater nutritional intake.[44,45] Longer survival time and better physical function were found 3 months post–ICU discharge in critically ill patients provided with adequate energy and nutrients.[46]

IMPLICATIONS FOR PRACTICE

Critically ill patients, especially at high nutrition risk, need to be fed sooner versus later but without overfeeding energy (ie, approximately 80% to 90% of calorie needs).[32] The use of enteral nutrition, especially when initiated early (ie, <48 hours from admission), is associated with significant reductions in infections and a trend toward reductions in mortality versus compared with delayed (after 48 hours) initiation of enteral nutrition in critically ill patients.[47–50] Enteral (as opposed to parenteral) nutrition also facilitates the maintenance of gastrointestinal tract tissues' integrity, structure, and function and helps reduce intestinal permeability and inflammation. Although disease severity moderates these beneficial effects, complications are more likely if energy (calories) and protein provisions are inadequate.[48] Benefits from enteral feedings are greatest when 80% or more of estimated energy (calorie) needs is provided.[44]

Multiple approaches are available to improve the adequacy of nutrient delivery to critically ill patients. The addition of intravenous amino acid infusions to enteral nutrition during the first week of ICU admission has been shown to improve protein balance in critically ill patients. The use of high protein (35% or more of energy) enteral nutrition products was also shown to help meet targeted protein needs of critically ill patients.[49] High-quality protein supplements also may be given to some patients receiving enteral nutrition or can be provided in quantities to solely meet individual protein prescription.[29] Substantial improvements in the provisions of energy (calories), protein, and other nutrients have been demonstrated in critically ill ICU patients with the use of nutrition protocols that base delivery of enteral nutrition on volume versus the standard approach, using rate.[29,40,41,51,52] Volume-based protocols set 24-hour goals versus hourly rates for the delivery of enteral feeds. With the use of volume-based protocols, interruptions in feeding from common issues, such as out-of-room diagnostic testing/imaging and return trips to the operating room, can be compensated by increased feeding rates. The higher rate compensates for the deficits that occurred secondary to enteral feeding disruptions and enables the delivery of prescribed amounts of energy (calories) and protein. Use of this 24-hour volume-based regimen, referred to as the Enhanced Protein-Energy Provision via the Enteral Route Feeding Protocol in Critically Ill Patients (PEP uP), was investigated in a repeated cross-sectional cluster randomized trial involving 18 ICUs throughout North America.[53] The findings showed significantly higher amounts of energy, protein, and other nutrients were provided with the use of this volume-based protocol versus the standard rate-based protocol.[40,41] (Note: information and education designed for nurses was developed along with bedside tools to meet learning needs and facilitate implementation of the PEP uP protocol.[53] Improvements in the provision of enteral nutrition are helping to ensure adequate protein and energy intakes are being achieved in critically ill patients. Studies are still needed, however, to address many unanswered questions.[32] The lower muscle protein synthesis response, for example, to increased amino acid concentrations (referred to as anabolic resistance) that is observed in healthy older adults needs to be considered and investigated in those who are critically ill.[6,54–56] Similarly, would bolus or intermittent feedings of load doses of protein, provided equally 3 times or 4 times per day, help to overcome the anabolic resistance and muscle full effects in critically ill patients and thus better stimulate muscle protein synthesis versus continuous feedings over an extended time period of the day?[6,55,57–61] Additionally, it is important to ensure that a patient's protein needs are also met during the post–ICU hospitalization stay when the catabolic phase of critical illness has diminished or is diminishing.[62]

Perhaps just as important to help correct the catabolic effects of illness on muscle and ICUAW is the need for ambulation and physical rehabilitation. Physical therapy can help enhance muscle protein synthesis. In the ICU, physical therapy has been shown in a small number of studies to improve muscle strength, physical function, and quality of life and to reduce length of ICU and hospital stays.[63] Similarly, and like physical therapy, also in need of more research is the use of electrical muscle stimulation in the ICU.[3] Physical therapy are important interventions to maintain muscle for the ICU patient, which in turn will improve physical function and psychological function. Physical therapy also may help to prevent cognitive decline and dementia.[17,18,64,65]

SUMMARY

Nurses play multiple essential roles in the care of critically ill patients in the ICU. Ensuring that patients meet their nutritional goals is one such role. Strict monitoring of the amounts of feeding is crucial. Finding methods to prevent interruption of enteral nutrition also is key. Working with a multidisciplinary team to have appropriate orders and maintain adequate nutrition corrects catabolic effects of muscle. Additionally, working with a multidisciplinary team to promote early ambulation, physical therapy, and electrical muscle stimulation is vital for nurses to oversee these important processes, thus helping to promote positive psychological, physical, and cognitive outcomes in critically ill patients.

REFERENCES

1. Monk DN, Plank LD, Franch-Arcas G, et al. Sequential changes in the metabolic response in critically injured patients during the first 25 days after blunt trauma. Ann Surg 1996;223(4):395–405.
2. Puthucheary ZA, Rawal J, McPhail M, et al. Acute skeletal muscle wasting in critical illness. JAMA 2013;310(15):1591–600.
3. Parry SM, El-Ansary D, Cartwright MS, et al. Ultrasonography in the intensive care setting can be used to detect changes in the quality and quantity of muscle and is related to muscle strength and function. J Crit Care 2015;30(5):1151.e9-14.
4. Plank LD, Hill GL. Similarity of changes in body composition in intensive care patients following severe sepsis or major blunt injury. Ann N Y Acad Sci 2000;904(1): 592–602.
5. Kortebein P, Ferrando A, Lombeida J, et al. Effect of 10 days of bed rest on skeletal muscle in healthy older adults. JAMA 2007;297(16):1772–4.

6. Paddon-Jones D, Sheffield-Moore M, Urban RJ, et al. Essential amino acid carbohydrate supplementation ameliorates muscle protein loss in humans during 28 days of bedrest. J Clin Endocrinol Metab 2004;89(9):4351–8.

7. Moore FA, Phillips SM, McClain CJ, et al. Nutrition support for persistent inflammation, immunosuppression, and catabolism syndrome. Nutr Clin Pract 2017; 32(suppl 1):121S–7S.

8. Kress JP, Hall JB. ICU-acquired weakness and recovery from critical illness. N Engl J Med 2014;370(17):1626–35.

9. Cruz-Jentoft AJ, Bahat G, Bauer J, et al. Writing Group for the European Working Group on sarcopenia in older people 2 (EWGSOP2), and the extended Groupfor EWGSOP2. Sarcopenia: revised European consensus on definition and diagnosis. Age Ageing 2019;48(1):16–31.

10. Herridge MS, Tansey CM, Matté A, et al. Canadian Critical Care Trials Group. Functional disability 5 years after acute respiratory distress syndrome. N Engl J Med 2011;364(14):1293–304.

11. Iwashyna TJ, Ely EW, Smith DM, et al. Long-term cognitive impairment and functional disability among survivors of severe sepsis. JAMA 2010;304(16):1787–94.

12. Janssen I, Heymsfield SB, Ross R. Low relative skeletal muscle mass (sarcopenia) in older persons is associated with functional impairment and physical disability. J Am Geriatr Soc 2002;50(5):889–96.

13. Hunt D, Gropper SS, Miller KA, et al. Prevalence of older adults with low muscle mass living in a residential continuing care retirement community in Florida. Clin Nurs Stud 2019;7(1):83–8.

14. Short KR, Nair KS. The effect of age on protein metabolism. Curr Opin Clin Nutr Metab Care 2000;3(1):39–44.

15. Lexell J. Human aging, muscle mass, and fiber type composition. J Gerontol A Biol Sci Med Sci 1995;50:11–6.

16. Jackson K, Hunt D, Chapa D, et al. Sarcopenia - a baby boomers dilemma for nurse practitioners to discover, diagnose, and treat. J Nurs Educ Pract 2018; 8(9):77–86.

17. Viscogliosi G, DiBernardo MG, Ettorre E, et al. Handgrip strength predicts longitudinal changes in clock drawing test performance. An observations study in a sample of older non-demented adults. J Nutr Health Aging 2017;21(5):593–6.

18. Fritz NE, McCarthy CJ, Adamo DE. Handgrip strength as a means of monitoring progression of cognitive decline – a scoping review. Ageing Res Rev 2017;35: 112–23.

19. Ochoa Gautier JB, Martindale RG, Rugeles SJ, Hurt RT, Taylor B, Heyland DK, McClave SA. How much and what type of protein should a critically ill patient receive. Nutr Clin Pract 2017;32(suppl 1):6S–14S.

20. Barker LA, Gout BS, Crowe TC. Hospitalized malnutrition: prevalence, identification, and impact on patients and the healthcare system. Int J Environ Res Public Health 2011;8(2):514–27.

21. Lim SI, Ong KC, Chan YH, et al. Malnutrition and its impact on cost of hospitalization, length of stay, readmission, and 3-year mortality. Clin Nutr 2012;31(3): 345–50.

22. Jensen GL, Mirtallo J, Compher C, et al, International Consensus Guideline Committee. Adult starvation and disease-related malnutrition: a proposal for etiology-based diagnosis in the clinical practice setting from the International Consensus Guideline Committee. JPEN J Parenter Enteral Nutr 2010;34(2):156–9.

23. Maciel L, Franzosi OS, Nunes DSL, et al. Nutritional risk screening 20002 cut off to identify high-risk is a good predictor of ICU mortality in critically ill patients. Nutr Clin Pract 2019;34(1):137–41.
24. Kondrup J. Nutritional-risk scoring systems in the intensive care unit. Curr Opin Clin Nutr Metab Care 2014;17(2):177–82.
25. Compher C, Chittams J, Sammarco T, et al. Greater nutrient intake is associated with lower mortality in western and eastern critically ill patients with low BMI: a multicenter, multinational observational study. JPEN J Parenter Enteral Nutr 2019;43(1):63–9.
26. McClave SA, Taylor BE, Martindale RG, et al. Guidelines for the provision and assessment of nutrition support therapy in the adult critically ill patient. Society of Critical Care Medicine (SCCM) and American Society for Parenteral and Enteral Nutrition (ASPEN). JPEN J Parenter Enteral Nutr 2016;40(2):159–211.
27. Canales C, Elsayes A, Yeh D, et al. Nutrition risk in critically ill versus the nutritional risk screening 2002: are they comparable for assessing risk of malnutrition in critically ill patients? JPEN J Parenter Enteral Nutr 2019;43(1):81–7.
28. Lee Z, Heyland DK. Determination of nutrition risk and status in critically ill patients: what are our considerations. Nutr Clin Pract 2019;34(1):96–111.
29. Heyland DK, Wejis PJM, Coss-Bu JA, et al. Protein delivery in the intensive care unit: optimal or suboptimal? Nutr Clin Pract 2017;31(1):58S–571S.
30. Heyland DK, Dhaliwal R, Jiang X, et al. Identifying critically ill patients who benefit the most from nutritional therapy: the development and initial validation of a novel risk assessment tool. Crit Care 2011;15(6):R268.
31. Parris M, Mourtzakis M. Assessment of skeletal muscle mass in critically ill patients. Considerations for the utility of computed tomography imaging and ultrasound. Curr Opin Clin Nutr Metab Care 2016;19(2):125–30.
32. Hurt RT, McClave SA, Martindale RG, et al. Summary points and consensus recommendations for the international protein summit. Nutr Clin Pract 2017;32(suppl 1):1425–515.
33. Fetterplace K, Deane AM, Tierney A, et al. Targeted full energy and protein delivery in critically ill patients: a pilot randomized controlled trial (FEED Trial). JPEN J Parenter Enteral Nutr 2018;42(8):1252–62.
34. Ferrie S, Allman-Farinelli M, Daley M, et al. Protein requirements in the critically ill: a randomized controlled trial using parenteral nutrition. JPEN J Parenter Enteral Nutr 2016;40(6):795–805.
35. Bauer JM, Verlaan S, Bautmans I, et al. Effects of vitamin D and leucine-enriched whey protein nutritional supplement on measures of sarcopenia in older adults, the PROVIDE Study: a randomized, double-blind, placebo-controlled trial. J Am Med Dir Assoc 2015;16(9):740–7.
36. Deutz NEP, Bauer JM, Barazzoni R, et al. Protein intake and exercise for optimal muscle function with aging: recommendations from the ESPEN Expert Group. Clin Nutr 2014;33(6):929–36.
37. Heyland DK, Schroter-Noppe D, Drover JW, et al. Nutrition support in the critical care setting: current practices in Canadian ICUs- opportunities for improvement. JPEN J Parenter Enteral Nutr 2003;27(1):74–83.
38. Jones NE, Dhaliwar R, Day AG, et al. Nutrition therapy in critical care setting: what is best achievable practice? Crit Care Med 2010;38(2):1–7.
39. DeWaele E, Spapen H, Honore PM, et al. Bedside calculation of energy expenditure does not guarantee adequate caloric prescription in long-term mechanically ventilated critically ill patients: a quality control study. ScientificWorldJournal 2012. https://doi.org/10.1100/2012/909564.

40. Heyland DK, Dhaliwal R, Lemieux ML, et al. Implementing the PEPuP protocol in critical care units in Canada: results of a multicenter quality improvement study. JPEN J Parenter Enteral Nutr 2015;39(6):698–706.
41. Heyland DK, Murch L, Cahill N, et al. Enhanced protein-energy provision via the enteral route feeding protocol in critically ill patients: results of a cluster randomized trial. Crit Care Med 2013;41(12):2743–53.
42. Nicolo M, Heyland DK, Cittams J, et al. Critical outcomes related to protein delivery in a critically ill population: a multicenter, multinational observation study. JPEN J Parenter Enteral Nutr 2016;40(1):46–51.
43. Compher C, Chittams J, Sammarco T, et al. Greater protein and energy intake may be associated with improved mortality in higher risk critically ill patients: a multicenter, multinational observational study. Crit Care Med 2017;45(2):156–63.
44. Alberda C, Gramlich L, Jones N, et al. The relationship between nutritional intake and clinical outcomes in critically ill patients: results of an international multicenter observational study. Intensive Care Med 2009;35(10):1728–37.
45. Wei X, Day AG, Quellette-Kuntz H, et al. The association between nutritional adequacy and long-term outcomes in critically ill patients requiring prolonged mechanical ventilation: a multicenter cohort study. Crit Care Med 2015;43(8): 1569–79.
46. McClave SA, Heyland DK. The physiologic response and associated clinical benefits from provision of early enteral nutrition. Nutr Clin Pract 2009;24(3):305–15.
47. Heyland DK, Stephens KE, Day AG, et al. The success of enteral nutrition and ICU-acquired infections: a multicenter observational study. Clin Nutr 2011; 30(2):148–55.
48. Doig GS, Heighes PT, Simpson F, et al. Early enteral nutrition, provided within 24 h of injury or intensive care unit admission, significantly reduces mortality in critically ill patients: a meta-analysis of randomized controlled trials. Intensive Care Med 2009;35(12):2018–27.
49. Liebau F, Sundström M, van Loon LJ, et al. Short-term amino acid infusion improves protein balance in critically ill patients. Crit Care 2015;19:106.
50. Hopkins B, Alberda C. Achieving protein targets in the ICU with a specialized enteral formula. Can J Diet Pract Res 2016;77(3):e1–2.
51. Taylor B, Brody R, Denmark R, et al. Improving enteral nutrition delivery through the adoption of the "Feed Early Enteral Diet adequately for Maximum Effect (FEED ME)" protocol in a surgical trauma ICU: a quality improvement review. Nutr Clin Pract 2014;29(5):639–48.
52. McClave SA, Saad MA, Esterle M, et al. Volume-based feeding in the critically ill patient. JPEN J Parenter Enteral Nutr 2015;39(6):707–12.
53. McCall M, Cahill N, Murch L, et al. Lessons learned from implementing a novel feeding protocol: results of a multicenter evaluation of educational strategies. Nutr Clin Pract 2014;29(4):510–7.
54. Moore DR, Churchward-Venne TR, Witard O, et al. Protein ingestion to stimulate myofibrillar protein synthesis requires greater relative protein intakes in healthy older versus younger men. J Gerontol A Biol Sci Med Sci 2015;70(1):57–72.
55. Martindale RG, Heyland DK, Rugeles SJ, et al. Protein kinetics and metabolic effects related to disease states in the intensive care unit. Nutr Clin Pract 2017; 32(1S):21S–9S.
56. Shad BJ, Thompson JL, Breen L. Does the muscle protein synthetic response to exercise and amino acid-based nutrition diminish with advancing age? A systematic review. Am J Physiol Endrocrinol Metab 2016;311(5):E803–17.

57. Bear DE, Hart N, Puthucheary Z. Continuous or intermittent feeding: pros and cons. Curr Opin Crit Care 2018;24(4):256–61.
58. Marik PE. Feeding critically ill patients the right "whey": thinking outside the box. A personal view. Ann Intensive Care 2015;5(1):51.
59. Bohe J, Low JFA, Wolfe RR, et al. Latency and duration of stimulation of human muscle protein synthesis during continuous infusion of amino acids. J Physiol 2001;532(2):575–9.
60. Loenneke JP, Loprinzi PD, Murphy CH, et al. Per meal dose and frequency of protein consumption is associated with lean mass and muscle performance. Clin Nutr 2016;35(6):1506–11.
61. Mamerow MM, Mettler JA, English KL, et al. Dietary protein distribution positively influences 24-h muscle protein synthesis in healthy adults. J Nutr 2014;144(6):876–80.
62. Ridley EJ, Parke RL, Davies AR, et al. What happens to nutrition intake in the post-intensive care unit hospitalization period? An observational cohort study in critically ill adults. JPEN J Parenter Enteral Nutr 2019;43(1):88–95.
63. Kayambu G, Boots R, Paratz J. Physical therapy for the critically ill in the ICU: a systematic review and meta-analysis. Crit Care Med 2013;41(6):1543–54.
64. Sternang O, Reynolds CA, Finkel D, et al. Grip strength and cognitive abilities: associations in old age. J Gerontol B Psychol Sci Soc Sci 2016;71(5):841–8.
65. Firth J, Stubbs B, Vancampfort D, et al. Grip strength is associated with cognitive performance in schizophrenia and the general population: a UK Biobank study of 476559 participants. Schizophr Bull 2018;44(4):728–36.

Impact of Early Mobilization in the Intensive Care Unit on Psychological Issues

Islande Joseph, BSN, RN*, Renee McCauley, MSN, RN, CCRN[1]

KEYWORDS

- Early mobilization • ICU • Psychosocial issues in the ICU
- Benefits of early mobilization • Change theory

KEY POINTS

- Early mobility improves outcomes in intensive care unit (ICU) patients.
- Early mobilization improves psychosocial issues in ICU patients.
- Change theory provides framework for early mobilization in ICU patients.

EARLY MOBILIZATION

The primary objective of any health care professional is to improve outcomes for patients. Overall, the anticipated result of such health care goals is to decrease the length of admissions and expedite safe releases from the hospital. In reality, the journey for critical care patients is burdened with increased risks of both foreseeable and some unexpected complications, which limit the ability to achieve such goals. Growing evidence suggests that neuromuscular disorders are responsible for an increase in both short-term and long-term physical morbidity in survivors of critical sickness.[1] Among possible risks factors, bed rest and its associated mechanisms may play a vital role in the pathogenesis of neuromuscular complications in critically ill patients. Early mobilization of these patients can help in the recovery of functional status and, therefore, improving patient outcomes. The purpose of this quality-improvement project was to test an intervention designed to improve early mobilization and decrease neuromuscular. The purpose of this article is to identify and define this nursing problem requiring change in the organization or unit, to determine the stakeholders involved in early mobilization, and to identify and discuss a proposed change to current mobilization practices. The impact of the change to the stakeholders and organization is

Disclosure Statement: The authors have nothing to disclose.
Medical Intensive Care Unit, Lee Memorial Hospital, Fort Myers, FL, USA
[1] Present address: 3741 Southwest 2nd Avenue, Cape Coral, FL 33914.
* Corresponding author. 11313 Pond Cypress Street, Fort Myers, FL 33913.
E-mail address: Islande.joseph@leehealth.org

explained and the role and leadership characteristics, skills, and competencies needed to implement the change described.

HISTORICAL BACKGROUND

Comparatively, histories of health system development have significantly changed over the years. Evidence shows that bed rest in critically ill patients was thought to be an aspect of recovery because it was believed that the preservation of energy would be helpful, especially for mechanically ventilated patients. During the late nineteenth century, early mobilization of sick patients was integrated into health care systems as a tool with many benefits, including improvements in muscle strength, functional mobility, and quality of life.[2] Early mobilization is defined as a series of intensive physical activities that starts within the 24 hours to 48 hours after a procedure or during an intensive care unit (ICU) admission.[3] Since the implementation of early mobilization in the health care setting, it has been linked to many positive outcomes among critically ill patients. According to Haris and Shahid,[4] prolonged periods of bedrest place critically ill patients at a higher risk for many complications, ranging from short-term impairments eg, neuromuscular weakness, increased time on mechanical ventilation, and longer ICU stays to long-term impairments in physical functioning. Such long-term physical impairments, along with impairments in cognition and mental health, are collectively termed post–intensive care syndrome. Early rehabilitative interventions, begun as soon as critically ill patients are deemed physiologically stable (ie, their clinical status is no longer declining), are beneficial to reducing patient complications. Such interventions frequently occur while patients are on mechanical ventilation and/or vasopressor infusions. Traditionally, patients are mobilized after, as opposed to during, their critical illness. For example, it is a common misconception that it is contraindicated to mobilize patients on vasopressors. With careful screening, such patients may be safely mobilized. Evidence shows early rehabilitation of ICU patients is both safe and feasible and also reduces hospital-acquired delirium and muscle weakness along with hospital length of stay.[5]

SYSTEM ISSUE

As discussed previously, the improvements and outcomes that have been seen are decreasing the effects of muscle atrophy from extended periods of immobility and increasing the ease of returning to a patient's baseline physical function as well as providing patients with opportunities to participate in and take ownership of their own recovery. All of these potential advantages of early mobility encourage a functional independence that positively affects a patient's emotional and psychological health, which in turn provides a more optimal environment for overall recovery and quality of life.[2]

Progressive mobility in critically ill/ICU patients has proved to be safe and beneficial. The implementation of the program into clinical care routines, however, can be challenging. According to Saunders,[6] some of the barriers of early mobilization are lack of knowledge, lack of staff and medical supplies, the complicated nature of mechanically intubated patients, sedation and delirium, multiples lines and tubes, and patient comorbidities. Nevertheless, incorporating staff teaching to combat these problems can be effective in successfully implementing mobility in the ICU patient population. When staffs are more aware of the process of early mobilization, they are able to provide better continuity and cohesiveness of care.

STAKEHOLDERS

The medical intensive care unit (MICU) hospital has 18 beds staffed with intensivist physicians; advanced registered nurse practitioners and physician assistants also are assigned to the unit. The registered nurse-to-patient ratio of 1:2 and 1 respiratory therapist are assigned with an assistant. One physical therapist (PT) and 1 occupational therapist (OT) are assigned on a rotating basis. Case involvement by PT and OT is dependent on a consultation request by a physician. In the MICU, bedrest is prescribed activity level in standard admission orders. There was no MICU guidelines for consultation or treatment by a PT or OT. Standard nursing care includes repositioning patients in bed every 2 hours and use of standardized pain and sedation scales (eg, Richmond Agitation-Sedation Scale), with a nurse-titrated sedation protocol. Standardized assessments for delirium in the MICU are not part of routine nursing care. Daily sedation reduction was per orders and usually addressed only as part of the preparation for intubating ventilated patients.

Achievement of early mobilization in critically ill patients requires coordination, commitment, and physical effort by the multidisciplinary team. proNurses must work to strengthen the long tradition of pulling together the many stakeholders within health care, such as the unit director, physicians, advanced providers, unit managers, staff nurses, PTs and OTs, pharmacists, case managers, bedside technicians, patients, and family members.[7] Although this tradition started with Florence Nightingale, any new nurses who identify their critical role in addressing the main issue of health care delivery at the bedside will ensure nursing enters into a collaborative relationship with other stakeholders at the organization. The experience of implementing an early mobility program in the MICU, in which the authors work, confirmed the efficacy of a program as well as the need for a multidisciplinary approach.

PROPOSED AND THEORY CHANGE

Experience confirms the applications of evidence-based therapies are notoriously difficult to integrate into practice. According to Messer and colleagues,[1] the theory of change is the step-by-step strategy for translating evidence into practice to include education, assessment, planning, and implementation. All components of this strategy must be employed to successfully affect change.

ACTION PLAN

The collaborative team gathers and summarizes evidence about immobility and mobilization. In order to strategize and implement best practice into the current bedside practice of mobilization within the organization/units, the team identifies the barriers to early mobilization and explains why the intervention is important. The information is then distributed in a concise manner, allowing all stakeholders to walk through the process and share opinions and potential dangers of the implementation. Input from multidisciplinary contributors can help ensure that mobility in critical ill patients/ICU becomes a regular practice.[6]

Perme and Chandrasekhar[8] designed a complete plan for early intervention of PT for ICU patients. The plan was designed with 4 phases and worked through the continuum of activity from passive range of motion to activities of daily living and ambulation. Phase 1 included patients who are critically ill with multiple medical problems and in an unstable conditioned at times. The goal in phase 1 is to start mobilization immediately on stabilization of a patient's medical condition. Therapeutic exercises were started keeping the patient in the supine position or with the head of the bed

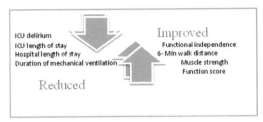

Fig. 1. Implementing the early mobilization protocol and increasing nursing knowledge improves patient outcomes through better management of personnel needed to complete transfers of patients being mobilized.

at the recommended degree of elevation. Phase 2 included patients whose overall medical condition and strength allowed standing activities with a walker, with the assistance of a therapist. Patients have to be able to follow simple commands and actively participate in therapy.

The focus of PT is to start walking, re-education, and functional training. Phase 3 is for patients who are able to accomplish limited walking with a walker and assistance. The PT in this phase focuses on the patient's ability to master transfer activities and start a progressive walking program to increase endurance. Phase 4 included patients who no longer require ventilator support or have been transferred out of the ICU. These patients have variable degrees of weakness and limitations but can participate in more intense therapy.

PROPOSAL RESULTS

Education is a vital component of implementing an early mobilization program in critically ill patients. Mobility teaching can be integrated into nursing education in an effort to help nurses overcome challenges and recognize the risks of immobility and benefits of mobilization in critically ill patients. Research indicates that by implementing this protocol and increasing nursing knowledge, patient outcomes improve through better management of personnel needed to complete transfers of patients being mobilized.[9] As a result, length of stay is decreased and, consequently, costs are reduced (**Fig. 1**).

LEADERSHIP SKILLS

In most critical care units, nurses are the chief providers of mobility for their patients. The unit leader can plan for and facilitate mandatory staff education. The mobilization protocol developed by the interdisciplinary team can then be used to educate unit staff on early mobilization and put in place the procedures necessary to successfully mobilize critically ill patients.[10] Although the authors were able to initiate a prescribed program of early mobilization in the MICU, there is an increased awareness of the benefits. The PT and OT team have started assessing patients for therapy as soon as they arrive in the unit; the critical team are consulting PT and OT much sooner than has been done in the past.

SUMMARY

In conclusion, integrating early mobilization activities into health care practice has been proved to prevent further muscle atrophy, hasten the return to baseline functional mobility, and improve overall quality of life in critically ill patients. Nonetheless, there are many factors that challenge the successful application of these interventions. Some of these factors are lack of knowledge, resources, and staff along with patient perception of care. Despite the many challenges that come with mobilizing the critically ill patient population, implementing protocols and teaching the promotion of early mobilization can make a big difference for health care professionals as well as patients. The complications associated with immobility have major negative pathophysiologic effects on patients, leading to increased lengths of stay and increased patient care costs. Evidence shows that early mobilization can prevent many of these complications and consequently improve patient outcomes. Initiation of a multidisciplinary team to address the problem of immobility can expedite patient recoveries and lead to the satisfaction of all stakeholders. Early mobilization is extremely beneficial to patients, which is why it is so important to work hard to ensure that it can be implemented effectively within the health care setting.

REFERENCES

1. Messer A, Comer L, Forst S. Implementation of a progressive mobilization program in a medical-surgical intensive care unit. Crit Care Nurse 2015;35(5):28–42.
2. Parry A. Importance of early mobilization in critical care patients. Br J Nurs 2016; 25(9):486–8.
3. Hopkins RO, Mitchell L, Thomsen GE, et al. Implementing a mobility program to minimize post-intensive care syndrome. AACN Adv Crit Care 2016;27(2): 187–203.
4. Harris CL, Shahid S. Physical therapy-driven quality improvement to promote early mobility in the intensive care unit. Proc (Bayl Univ Med Cent) 2014;27(3): 203–7.
5. Klein K, Mulkey M, Bena JF, et al. Clinical and psychological effects of early mobilization in patients treated in a neurologic ICU: a comparative study. Crit Care Med 2015;43(4):865–73.
6. Saunders CB. Preventing secondary complications in trauma patients with implementation of multidisciplinary mobilization team. J Trauma Nurs 2015;22(3): 170–5.
7. Bassett RD, Vollman KM, Brandwene L, et al. Integrating a multidisciplinary mobility program into intensive care practice (IMMPTP): A multicenter collaborative. Intensive Crit Care Nurs 2014;28:88–97.
8. Perme C, Chandrashekar R. Early mobility and walking program for patients in intensive care units: creating a standard of care. Am J Crit Care 2009;18: 212–21. https://doi.org/10.4037/ajcc200959.
9. Amidei C. Measurement of physiologic responses to mobilization in critically ill adults. Intensive Crit Care Nurs 2012;28(2):58–72.
10. Needham DM, Korupolu R, Zanni JM, et al. Early physical medicine and rehabilitation for patients with acute respiratory failure: a quality improvement project. Arch Phys Med Rehabil 2010;91(4):536–42.

Postintensive Care Syndrome

Sharon E. Bryant, DNP, ACNP-BC, RN, MSN*, Kathryn McNabb, DNP, AGACNP, RN, MSN

KEYWORDS

- Intensive care • Syndrome • Critical care • Delirium • Immobility • Caregiver burden
- PTSD

KEY POINTS

- Intensive care unit (ICU) syndrome can affect cognitive, psychological, and/or physical domains.
- Early prevention measures can be incorporated in the ICU that potentially reduce the severity of symptoms.
- Symptoms related to ICU syndrome may remain for years after hospital discharge and are defined as postintensive care syndrome.
- Caregiver strain can coexist with all levels of ICU and should be frequently evaluated by all providers.

INTRODUCTION

More than 5 million patients are admitted to the intensive care unit (ICU) each year.[1] ICU admissions are associated with higher illness acuity due to life-threatening illness and require multiple life-saving interventions. Recent interest has focused on the short-term and long-term outcomes of intensive care survivors and their families. Patients who survive critical illness often have multifaceted needs that require thorough evaluation and targeted interventions posthospitalization. ICU survivors have higher rates of mortality and increased health care utilization postdischarge.[2]

Intensive care syndrome is defined as a cluster of symptoms that are unique to the ICU environment, including alterations in cognition, psychiatric manifestations, and physical ability. Onset of alterations in cognition and psychological and physical impairments can start to occur 24 to 48 hours after admission and the aftereffects can be seen in ICU survivors up to 5 years and beyond after hospital discharge. These continued impairments after hospital discharge include deficits in cognition and executive functioning, depression, anxiety, posttraumatic stress disorder (PTSD), and

Disclosure: The authors have nothing to disclose.
Vanderbilt University School of Nursing, 461 21st Avenue South, Nashville, TN 37214, USA
* Corresponding author.
E-mail address: Sharon.bryant@vanderbilt.edu

cognitive impairment, all of which make up the what is now termed postintensive care syndrome (PICS).[3,4] Families and caregivers may also suffer from a form of PICS termed PICS-family (PICS-F). Frequently these symptoms are not recognized by providers and leave caregivers without needed support.[5] This article discusses the neuropathogenesis of intensive care syndrome, including common assessment findings and current trends for management in the ICU, post-ICU discharge, and after hospital discharge. Owing to the profound impact of ICU syndrome on the family unit, issues related to caregiver burden are often overlooked and this is also discussed.

EPIDEMIOLOGY

The increasing prevalence of critical care illnesses combined with improved care and reduced mortality associated with ICU admission has led to increased numbers of ICU survivors.[6] Due to the neuropsychological and functional impairments associated with PICS, it is now recognized as a public health burden.[4] As ICU providers push the limitations of survival, many of these survivors suffer ICU deficits in 1 of 3 general domains: physical, cognitive, and psychiatric. The constellation of sequelae has been termed intensive care syndrome and is not only exhibited in critical illness survivors but also in their families and caregivers.[7] Studies conclude that most survivors of critical illness suffer some form of ICU syndrome and PICS after ICU discharge. One study evaluated a cohort of survivors at 3 months and 12 months, and estimated that 64% of survivors suffered from PICS at 3 months after hospital discharge and 56% suffered from PICS at 12 months. Fewer than 20% of all survivors have more than 1 reported impairment. The most frequently reported impairment is altered cognition, with more than 25% of all ICU survivors suffering from some form of cognitive impairment after hospital discharge, followed by depression, then physical disability.[8] The risk of developing psychological disabilities ranges greatly (1%–62%) and is specifically manifested as depression, anxiety, and PTSD.[4]

FACTORS CONTRIBUTING TO THE DEVELOPMENT OF INTENSIVE CARE UNIT SYNDROME
Cognitive Impairment

Risk factors for cognitive impairment associated with ICU syndrome include ICU delirium, severity of illness, and a prior history of cognitive insults. Delirium is the most common problem associated with ICU admission. Common factors for the development of delirium include genetics, illness severity, environment, and medications.[9] Additional risk factors for cognitive impairment include female gender, lower education level, preexisting disability, and use of sedation and analgesia in the ICU.[4]

Termed ICU psychosis, ICU delirium has been defined as a neurobehavioral syndrome resulting from an imbalance in neurotransmitter synthesis, function, or availability. Neurotransmitter imbalance may occur in a constellation of patterns and result in a spectrum of clinical features ranging from increased agitation and hyperactivity to somnolence and withdrawal. Variation in occurrence rates of delirium has been seen in institutions and institutional critical care units, and can be attributed to varying patient populations, illness acuity distribution, and screening tools.[9] The average length of a delirium episode ranges between 2 and 7 days; however, in some cases, delirium can last for weeks.[10] Delirium is the most common surgical complication in older adults, having an incidence of 15% to 25% after elective surgery and upwards of 50% after major surgical procedures, including cardiac surgery.[11,12] After age 65 years, the risk of delirium increases 2% with each additional year of life.[13] Delirium incidence approaches 90% when older adults progress to palliative care settings.[14]

Illness Severity

Conditions such as septic shock, metabolic acidosis, and polytrauma precipitate an acute inflammatory response, which can lead to the development of intensive care syndrome.[9,13] Mechanical ventilation and increased procedure requirements suggest increased complexity of illness and can decrease cognition.[15] Increased illness severity results in increased environmental stimuli. Environmental factors have long been shown to affect the risk of delirium development. Dark rooms, continual noise, and frequent disruptions are proven risk factors for delirium.[16] Medications, particularly benzodiazepines and opioids, have a dose-dependent risk associated with delirium development. In essence, any medication that crosses the blood–brain barrier can put a patient at risk for delirium.[17,18]

Psychiatric Illness

Anxiety, depression, and PTSD are the most common psychiatric disturbances associated with PICS. Risk factors associated with the development of psychiatric manifestations include female gender, low socioeconomic status, unemployment, preexisting psychiatric illness, and personality disorder. ICU management strategies contributing to psychiatric manifestations include prolonged mechanical ventilation time, use of antipsychotics or sedation, and restraints.[19]

Physical Weakness

The term ICU-acquired illness describes the generalized muscle weakness found in patients recovering from critical illness. These patients have a constellation of symptoms, including muscle weakness, decreased strength, and various pain syndromes. There is no identifiable cause for these myopathic findings; however, muscle wasting due to atrophy and a net catabolic balance due to high levels of protein breakdown and decreased muscle protein synthesis are both thought to contribute.[17] Patients with hemodynamic instability are not generally candidates for physical therapy and are not seen by a therapist. Conversely, many inpatient therapists do not receive adequate training on how to provide therapy to critically ill patients. In many cases, therapy is not performed until supportive measures, such as mechanical ventilation or vasopressor therapy, are discontinued and the patient has transferred to a stepdown floor.

PREVENTION AND MANAGEMENT OF INTENSIVE CARE UNIT SYNDROME

Pain in the ICU is experienced by more than 50% of all ICU patients. Procedures, immobility, and mechanical ventilation are main contributors to pain.[17,19] The gold standard for pain assessment is patient reporting; however, many patients are unable to report their pain owing to cognitive or physical limitations. In addition to the traditional Wong-Baker Faces used in years past, more effective clinical tools have been validated to screen pain in the ICU, including the Behavioral Pain Scale and the Critical-Pain Observation Tool. Each tool evaluates behavioral patterns of patients, providing a quantitative measurement for pain.[20] Routine administration of pain medication is recommended for pain prevention and management.[17] Uncontrolled pain syndromes can lead to anxiety, fear, and the development of delirium, which decreases the progression of ventilator weaning.[21]

Oversedation contributes to the development of cognitive and psychiatric symptoms. Current ICU guidelines recommend decreased use of sedation for ventilated patients. Daily assessment using spontaneous breath trials are recommended to decrease the length of time that patients require invasive ventilation.[21]

Targeted patient sedation should be used as needed for purposeful sedation. Targeted sedation can be monitored by using tools such as the Richmond Agitation Sedation Scale (RASS), Riker Sedation Agitation Scale, or the Ramsay Sedation Scale.[22] The RASS tool has shown superior performance in measuring sedation depth.[22] Individualized sedation and analgesia management is critical in the prevention of cognitive impairment, such as confusion and delirium, and also allows for pain relief to increase mobility. Benzodiazepines have been linked to increased risk of delirium, whereas dexmedetomidine is associated with decreased rates of delirium and shorter ventilator days.[22]

An estimated 25% of all critically ill patients develop some form of delirium within 24 hours of hospital admission with studies reporting almost 90% of all patients manifesting some degree of delirium at some point during an ICU admission. Difficulty in recognizing simple confusion patterns during bedside interaction resulted in underrecognition of delirium by medical staff.[23,24] Preventative strategies have demonstrated a positive impact on preventing long-term functional disabilities associated with PICS.[4] Recommendations for frequent and routine screening of all ICU patients have led to earlier identification of delirium patterns. Tools such as the Confusion Assessment Method and Intensive Care Delirium Screening Checklist are most frequently used for screening delirium.[23,24]

Environmental modifications are effective in decreasing the risk of delirium. Dark rooms, continual noise, and frequent disruptions are proven risk factors for delirium and should be avoided. Pharmacologic management of delirium includes minimizing the use of anticholinergics, opioids, and sedating medications.[25] Haloperidol (Haldol) has shown effectiveness in the prevention of delirium symptoms and is recommended for short-term use only.[26] Melatonin has shown to be effective in the prevention of delirium by helping to regulate sleep–wake cycles.[27] Additional strategies to prevent PICS include avoiding hypoglycemia and hypoxemia, and ICU diaries maintained by family members and health care providers. These interventions have been shown to reduce symptoms associated with PTSD.[4]

The effects of prolonged immobility include myopathy and atrophy of muscles, resulting in musculoskeletal deconditioning. Patients with prolonged immobility can lose up to 2% of lean body mass per day, resulting in poor balance and coordination, along with joint stiffness.[28] Lack of early mobility occurs for several reasons. This can be as a result of provider and nursing perceptions that the patient is too sick to be active. It can also be due to challenges between nursing and multidisciplinary therapy services to coordinate patient mobility. Creating a new culture that focuses on early mobility and activity has shown to improve functional ability and possibly prevent ICU syndrome.[29,30] Physical activity that targets cardiopulmonary, musculoskeletal, and neurologic systems performed at least 20 minutes per day can reduce the length of ICU stay.[31] Early referral for rehabilitation has a positive impact on short-term physical recovery and should be made during the early stages of recovery to allow for evaluation of the patient by both the facility and the insurer for acceptance.[29]

Incorporation of family members and caregivers into the patient treatment plan has evolved. Many ICU settings now have a modified open visitation policy, allowing family and friends to visit the patient at will. Open communication of diagnoses, necessary procedures, and plans of care allow for participation in decision-making and expression of patient wishes and concerns. Various studies have shown that added family presence at the patient bedside does not increase stress on the health care team and does not interfere with the implementation of medical care.[32] Education and communication with family members and caregivers has shown to decrease ICU days, promote family conferences and collaboration with providers, and allow for quicker transfer to supportive services such as palliative care. It is essential for medical staff to remain sensitive to the impact that ICU admission has on families and the patient's support system. Listening to family concerns and suggestions, and recognizing individual coping mechanisms for individual family members and caregivers, can help guide conversations about the patient illness trajectory and about when to call on multidisciplinary support persons such as chaplains to engage in family and caregiver support strategies.[33] Screening tools may be useful for both establishing a baseline and continued monitoring in one or more of the PICS domains. Examples of these tools are listed in **Box 1**.[34,35]

POSTINTENSIVE CARE TRANSITION

Recognition of ICU syndrome is necessary beyond the critical care unit. Discharge locations for ICU patients include hospital stepdown or general care wards, skilled nursing, inpatient rehabilitation, and long-term acute care hospitals. Care transition during the transfer process allows for adequate transfer of information for continuing providers. The routine use of screening tools may also be helpful in continuing to monitor the continued symptoms of ICU symptoms as they relate to the post-ICU time period. Screening tools such as the Short Form Health Survey (SF)-12 questionnaire (a modified version of the SF-36) have shown benefit to assessing health care–related quality of life.[36] The Healthy Aging Brain Center Monitor is a 27-item self-report questionnaire used to evaluate cognitive, functional, and psychological functioning of ICU survivors. It is used for patients who score greater than 17 on the Mini-Mental State Examination (MMSE).[35]

Box 1
Validated screening tools for intensive care unit and postintensive care unit syndromes

Cognitive

- Folstein Mini-Mental State Examination (MMSE)
- Trail Making Test (A and B)
- Montreal Cognitive Assessment
- Digit Span Memory Test

Psychological

- Geriatric Depression Scale (GDS)-30
- Patient Health Questionnaire (PHQ)-9
- Posttraumatic Stress Symptoms Checklist (PTSS)-10
- General Anxiety Disorder (GAD)-7
- Hospital Anxiety and Depression Scale (HADS)
- Primary Care PTSD Screen (PC-PTSD)

Physical Ability

- Physical Self-Maintenance Scale (PSMS)
- Lawton Instrumental Activities of Daily Living Scale
- Katz Index of Independence in Activities of Daily Living
- Nutritional Health Checklist

In many scenarios, the fallout of ICU syndrome is left for management by long-term and primary care providers (PCPs) in a variety of settings. Post-ICU clinics were established to improve cost-effectiveness of care and reduce delivery of fragmented care. Tangible outcomes of post-ICU clinics for patients have included counseling of medications currently prescribed, guidance on prognosis of diseases acquired during admission, and treatment of functional rehabilitative needs of the patient postdischarge.[37] Repeated discussion of ICU and post-ICU syndromes with family members and caregivers during ICU admission help facilitate comprehension of potential post-ICU needs.[2]

Transitional care programs (TCPs) use a multidisciplinary approach to follow older patients after discharge home and facilitate communication between patients and their PCP. TCPs have shown decreases in postdischarge complications, as well as hospital readmission rates.[38,39] Participation in follow-up clinics, as well as revisiting the ICU, have proven beneficial in helping patients recall and process their inpatient stay.[40] Specific evaluations are based on patient's physical function deficits; medication management with reconciliation and counseling; cognitive function with targeted psychotherapy; and mood by screening for depression, anxiety, and PTSD. Additionally, driving and return to work are discussed during initial appointments.[2]

Common post-ICU complications managed outside the ICU include myopathy, chronic pain syndromes (eg, neuropathy and paresthesia), shortness of breath, reduced appetite, depression, anxiety, and insomnia. Despite the common cause of PICS, these complications warrant additional outpatient evaluation and continued management. Anemias are common owing to blood loss, as well as bone marrow suppression from ICU-related medications.[28] Metabolic bone disease related to steroid use, prolonged immobility, and malnutrition may require both nutritional and osteoporosis screening. Patients requiring prolonged mechanical ventilation may require tracheostomy placement to promote ventilator weaning. Tracheal stenosis and fistula formation are rare; however, if recognized, these may require referral to surgical or pulmonary specialties.[41,42]

Patients may suffer from psychological and cognitive deficits for years post-ICU discharge. The lack of acute symptom onset combined with a vague timeline of symptom continuation or progression often results in a lack of deficit identification by providers. Sexual dysfunction may also occur either concurrently or separate from PTSD symptoms; however, a strong correlation exists between sexual dysfunction and PTSD. Symptoms such as lack of desire, performance issues, and physical limitation during intercourse are common complaints.[43] Depression is most common in patients with acute lung injury requiring prolonged ventilation. Patients with delirium have cognitive issues with memory recall, which can lead to increased anxiety levels. Cognitive impairment and sleep disorders may also be present, which may lead to prolonged unemployment or delay in return to work. Social isolation may occur as a result of 1 more of these complications and should be monitored in both patients and caregivers.[44]

CAREGIVER BURDEN OF POSTINTENSIVE CARE SYNDROME

Having a loved one in the ICU can be stressful and intimidating for family members and caregivers. Patients requiring mechanical ventilation, life-saving procedures, and expert consultation are receiving constant care throughout their admission with plans of care quickly changing. Family members may find themselves in role reversal from being placed in situations in which they are unexpectedly the decision-makers and may rely on other providers for final decisions. Fear of death or permanent disability, unplanned financial burden, and general uncertainty may lower the threshold of how family members and caregivers effectively deal with these concerns. Ranges of emotion from anger, grief, despair, crying, laughing, and guilt may be felt along the admission continuum. When these stressors are combined with constant noise of medical equipment and medical technology interface, it is easy for families to lose themselves in the constant whirlwind of the ICU. This loss of self-need can further result in maladaptive coping strategies, which may manifest during the patient's hospitalization or after discharge.[5,45]

Common psychological symptoms of PICS-F include depression and anxiety.[46] Depression is the most common symptom experienced, followed by anxiety, acute stress disorder, and PTSD. Impaired sleep habits both during the ICU stay and after discharge correlated with acute impairments and maladaptive coping. Hospital-related factors, including limited visiting times, severe illness, and lack of perceived communication by health care personnel, also played a role in the development of PICS-F. Additional risk factors for PICS-F are listed in **Box 2**.[5,46] Caregivers may not always state their frustrations or stress, shifting the burden of caregiver management to the outpatient provider to recognize and to provide resources for support.[5] Questionnaires such as the Zarit Burden Interview give insight to the degree of caregiver burden and may be used in the clinic setting. Interventions such as support groups and respite care provide caregiver holidays, allowing for individual self-care. Ineffective coping by a caregiver can lead to the mistreatment, abuse, or neglect of the patient, and should be immediately reported to local authorities.[45]

Standardization is needed to appropriately summate all reported burdens of PICS-F, as well as appropriately define caregiver burden. A summative review is needed that details all reported burdens and the associated impact on caregivers so, optimally, they can receive care if needed.[47] Studies have evaluated and compared the needs for medical staff and family members during ICU admissions and have found that the needs of each group vary. Nurses are trained to focus on the needs of the patient and, therefore, may not pay close attention to the needs of the family. Furthermore, families with maladaptive coping strategies may inadvertently push away medical staff by making inflammatory or accusatory criticisms regarding the patient's care. Both healthcare providers and family members want the best care for the patient however differences do exist with the perception of patient needs.[48] Families also want know specific factual details regarding patient care, interventions, and prognosis. Honest communication was key to families feeling engaged and aware of current situations. Nurses did not share the emotional needs of the families and thought it most important

---

Box 2
Risk factors for caregiver-related postintensive care syndrome

Female gender

Spousal caregiving

Illness severity of patient

Communication with hospital personnel

Preexisting history of mental illness

Low socioeconomic status

Low level of education

Caregiving greater than 100 hours per month

Lack of resources and support

to be aware of their loved one's ever-changing plan of care.[17] Appreciation of these differences can provide insight into navigating situational occurrences with families and caregivers during their ICU experience.

SUMMARY

Intensive care syndrome is defined as new or worsening impairments in physical, cognitive, or mental health status arising during critical illness. ICU syndrome extending beyond ICU discharge is called PICS and may persist for months to years after hospitalization.[3,4] As the long-term effects of critical illness are elucidated, health care facilities must develop and implement effective interventions to reduce incidence of incomplete recovery.[29] Both postintensive care survivors and family members suffer from varied impairments, including mental health deficits, cognitive impairments, and physical dysfunction, which are present both during ICU admission and after ICU discharge. These deficits have a negative impact on quality of life and can result in long-term disability. Targeted cognitive, psychiatric, and rehabilitative initiatives are effective at improving outcomes and enhancing quality of life for critically-ill patients posthospitalization.[2] Long-term outcomes research is needed to definitely evaluate the use of post-ICU clinics and their effectiveness at mortality reduction.[37]

REFERENCES

1. Needham DM, Davidson J, Cohen H, et al. Improving long-term outcomes after discharge from intensive care unit: report from a stakeholders' conference. Crit Care Med 2012;40:502–9.
2. Sevin CM, Bloom SL, Jackson JC, et al. Comprehensive care of ICU survivors: development and implementation of an ICU recovery center. J Crit Care 2018; 46:141–8.
3. McPeake J, Mikkelsen ME. The evolution of post intensive care syndrome. Crit Care Med 2018;46(9):1551–2.
4. Rawal G, Yadav S, Kumar R. Post-intensive care syndrome: an overview. J Transl Int Med 2017;5(2):90–2.
5. Aldeman R, Tmanova L, Delgado D, et al. Caregiver burden: a clinical review. JAMA 2014;311(10):1052–60.
6. Iwashyna TJ, Cooke CR, Wunsch H, et al. Population burden of long-term survivorship after severe sepsis in older Americans. J Am Geriatr Soc 2012;60: 1070–7.
7. Jones C, Humphris GM, Griffiths RD. Psychological morbidity following critical illness - the rationale for care after intensive care. Clin Intensive Care 1998;9: 199–205.
8. Marra A, Pandharipande PP, Girard TD, et al. Co-occurrence of post-intensive care syndrome problems among 406 survivors of critical illness. Crit Care Med 2018;46:1393–401.
9. Ouimet S, Riker R, Bergeon N, et al. Subsyndromal delirium in the ICU: evidence for a disease spectrum. Intensive Care Med 2007;33:1007–13.
10. Zaal I, Tekatli H, van der Kooi A, et al. Classification of daily mental status in critically ill patients for research purposes. J Crit Care 2015;30:375–80.
11. Marcantonio ER. Delirium in hospitalized older adults. N Engl J Med 2017;377: 1456–66.
12. Marcantonio ER. Postoperative delirium: a 76 year-old woman with delirium following surgery. JAMA 2012;308:73–81.

13. Pandharipande P, Shintani A, Peterson J, et al. Lorazepam is an independent risk factor for transitioning to delirium in intensive care unit patients. Anesthesiology 2006;104:21–6.
14. Inouye SK, Westendorp RG, Saczynski JS. Delirium in elderly people. Lancet 2014;383:911–22.
15. Almeida I, Soares M, Bozza F. The impact of acute brain dysfunction in the outcomes of mechanically ventilated cancer patients. PLoS One 2014;9:e85332.
16. Van Rompaey B, Elseviers M, Schuurmans M, et al. Risk factors for delirium in intensive care patients: a prospective study. Crit Care Med 2009;13:R77.
17. Barr J, Fraser GL, Puntillo K, et al. Clinical practice guidelines for the management of pain, agitation, and delirium in adult patients in the intensive care unit. Crit Care Med 2013;41:263–306.
18. Bear DE, Puthucheary ZA, Hart N. Early feeding during critical illness. Lancet Respir Med 2013;2(1):15–7.
19. Desai SV, Law TJ, Needham DM. Long-term complications of critical care. Crit Care Med 2011;39:371–9.
20. Gélinas C, Fillion L, Puntillo KA, et al. Validation of the critical-care pain observation tool in adult patients. Am J Crit Care 2006;15:420–7.
21. Puntillo K, Pasero C, Li D, et al. Evaluation of pain in ICU patients. Chest 2009; 135:1069–74.
22. Reissen R, Pech R, Trankle P, et al. Comparison of the Ramsay score and the Richmond Agitation-Sedation Scale for the measurement of sedation depth. Crit Care 2012;16(Suppl 1):326.
23. Brummel NE, Vasilevskis EE, Han JH, et al. Implementing delirium screening in the intensive care unit: secrets to success. Crit Care Med 2013;41(9):2196–208.
24. Hussein ME, Hirst S, Salyers V. Factors that contribute to underrecognition of delirium by registered nurses in acute care settings: a scoping review of the literature to explain this phenomenon. J Clin Nurs 2014;24:906–15.
25. Khan BA, Perkins AJ, Campbell NL, et al. Pharmacological management of delirium in the intensive care unit: a randomized pragmatic clinical trial. J Am Geriatr Soc 2019. https://doi.org/10.1111/jgs.15781.
26. Zayed Y, Barbarawi M, Kheiri B, et al. Haloperidol for the management of delirium in adult intensive care unit patients: a systematic review and meta-analysis of randomized controlled trials. J Crit Care 2019;50:280–6.
27. Abbasi S, Farsaei S, ghasemi D, et al. Potential role of exogenous melatonin supplement in delirium prevention in critically ill patients: a double blind randomized pilot study. Iran J Pharm Res 2018;17(4):1571–80.
28. Volk B, Grassi F. Treatment of the post-ICU patient in an outpatient setting. Am Fam Physician 2009;79(6):459–64.
29. Fuke R, Hifumi T, Kondo Y, et al. Early rehabilitation to prevent postintensive care syndrome in patients with critical illness: a systematic review and meta-analysis. BMJ 2017. https://doi.org/10.1136/bmjopen-2017-019998.
30. Makic MB. Rethinking mobility and intensive care patients. J Perianesth Nurs 2015;30:151–2.
31. Nordon-Craft A, Moss M, Quan D, et al. Intensive care unit acquired weakness: implications for physical therapist management. Phys Ther 2012;92:1494–506.
32. Jabre P, Belpomme V, Azoulay E, et al. Family presence during cardiopulmonary resuscitation. N Engl J Med 2013;368:1008–18.
33. Curtis JR, Engelberg RA, Wenrich MD, et al. Missed opportunities during famiy conferences about end-of-life care in the intensive care unit. Am J Respir Crit Care Med 2005;171:844–9.

34. Milton A, Brück E, Schandl A, et al. Early psychological screening of intensive care unit survivors: a prospective cohort study. Crit Care 2017;17:273.

35. Wang S, Allen D, Perkins A, et al. Validation of a new clinical too for post-intensive care syndrome. Am J Crit Care 2019;28(1):10–8.

36. Venni A, Ioia F, Laviola S, et al. Clinical utility of a structured program to reduce the risk of health-related quality of life impairment after discharge from intensive care unit: a real world experience. Crit Care Res Pract 2018. https://doi.org/10.1155/2018/3838962.

37. Teixeira C, Rosa RG. Post-intensive care outpatient clinic: is it feasible and effective? A literature review Ambulatório pós-unidade de terapia intensiva: é viável e efetivo? Uma revisão da literatura. Rev Bras Ter Intensiva 2018;30(1):98–111.

38. Naylor MD, Brooten D, Campbell R, et al. Comprehensive discharge planning and home follow-up of hospitalized elders: a randomized clinical trial. JAMA 1999;7:613–20.

39. Naylor MD, Aiken LH, Kurtzman ET, et al. The importance of transitional care in achieving health reform. Health Aff 2011;30(4):746–54.

40. Hanifa AL, Glaeemose AO, Laursen BS. Picking up the pieces: qualitative evaluation of follow-up consultations post intensive care admission. Intensive Crit Care Nurs 2018;48:85–91.

41. Scalise P, Prunk SR, Healy D, et al. The incidence of tracheoarterial fistula in patients with chronic tracheostomy tubes: a retrospective study of 544 patients in a long-term care facility. Chest 1998;114(4):1122–8.

42. Zias N, Chroneou A, Tabba MK, et al. Post tracheostomy and post intubation tracheal stenosis: report of 31 cases and review of the literature. BMC Pulm Med 2008;8(18). https://doi.org/10.1186/1471-2466-8-18.

43. Griffiths J, Gager M, Alder N, et al. Self-reported based study of the incidence and associations of sexual dysfunction in survivors of intensive care treatment. Intensive Care Med 2006;32(3):445–51.

44. Griffiths J, Fortune G, Barber V, et al. The prevalence of post-traumatic stress disorder in survivors of ICU treatment: a systematic review. Intensive Care Med 2007;33(9):1506–18.

45. Parks SM, Movielli KD. A practical guide to caring for caregivers. Am Fam Physician 2000;62(12):2613–20.

46. Serrano P, You NP, Kheir MD, et al. Aging and post-intensive care syndrome-family: a critical need for geriatric psychiatry. Am J Geriatr Psychiatry 2018. https://doi.org/10.1016/j.jagp.2018.12.

47. van Beusekom I, Bakhshi-Raiez F, de Keizer NF, et al. Reported burden on informal caregivers of ICU survivors: a literature review. Crit Care 2016;20:16.

48. Shorofi SA, Jannati Y, Moghaddam HR, et al. Psychosocial needs of families of intensive care patients: perceptions of nurses and families. Niger Med J 2016; 57(1):10–8.

Posttraumatic Stress Syndrome and Implications for Practice in Critical Care Nurses

Garrett Salmon, DNP, MS, BSN, APRN, CRNA*,
Angela Morehead, DNP, FNP-BC, RN

KEYWORDS

- Posttraumatic stress disorder • Nurse compassion fatigue • Resilience
- Nurse burnout • Nurse anxiety or depression • Critical care nursing

KEY POINTS

- Discuss the prevalence of posttraumatic stress disorder (PTSD) in critical care nurses.
- Identify contributing factors and consequences of PTSD in critical care nurses.
- Explain resilience and how this prevents the development of PTSD in critical care nurses.

INTRODUCTION

Nursing care is a critical constituent of the health care system in the United States. It is imperative that the nurse workforce remain as capable and robust as possible to meet the ongoing needs of patients nationwide. The US health care system is currently experiencing a critical shortage of competent nurses to meet the growing needs of patient care.[1] Lack of qualified and capable nurses is a problem that is expected to worsen over time. At present, the turnover rates among nurses in the United States health care system ranges from 15.8% to 30.5%.[2] This high attrition rate is particularly disconcerting to nursing staff in critical care units. High turnover rates can lead to increases in sentinel events, affecting increases in patient mortality and morbidity.[3] It is also important to note that the high turnover of critical care nurses can contribute to work-related stress, increased cost of training, and decreased satisfaction with the work environment. Critical care nursing is encased within a high-stress setting. Repeated exposure to extreme stressors and the inability to adjust to this challenging

Disclosure Statement: The authors have nothing to disclose.
Nursing, Middle Tennessee State University, 1301 East Main Street, MTSU Box 81, Murfreesboro, TN 37132, USA
* Corresponding author.
E-mail address: Garrett.Salmon@mtsu.edu

milieu may result in the development of significant psychological disorders such as symptoms of posttraumatic stress disorder (PTSD) in some nurses.[4] Therefore, the development of PTSD may play a significant role in the high rate of critical care nurses leaving the profession.

Exploring the relationship of PTSD, job satisfaction, and the shortage of nurses in the critical care nursing is of vital importance. This exploration must include attention to the prevalence of PTSD in critical care nurses, and investigation of contributing factors and the consequences of the problem if it continues. Once these factors have been identified, approaches and strategies that may decrease or prevent PTSD in critical care nurses must be examined and assessed to combat this alarming trend.

WHAT IS POSTTRAUMATIC STRESS DISORDER?

When discussing the importance of PTSD as it relates to critical care nurses, it is important to define and explore what PTSD is, so that one can see how this psychological disorder is identified and diagnosed in at-risk persons. PTSD is a psychiatric disorder that can occur in people who have experienced or witnessed a traumatic event such as a natural disaster, a serious accident, a terrorist act, war or combat, or rape or other violent personal assault.[5] People with PTSD have intense, disturbing thoughts and feelings related to their experience that last long after the traumatic event has ended.[5] In critical care nurses, it is easy to understand, given the responsibilities and duties they must perform, that the occurrence of this psychological phenomenon is a significant risk. Critical care nurses are repeatedly exposed to high-intensity events and stressors that are common in daily clinical practice. These events include cardiopulmonary resuscitation, caring for critically ill patients who require end-of-life care or life support while having their lives artificially prolonged, addressing end-of-life issues and postmortem care with patient families, and many other emotionally volatile situations.[4]

If a nurse has PTSD, the diagnosis can cause a significant negative impact on job performance and quality of life. People who have PTSD may relive the event through flashbacks or nightmares; they may feel sadness, fear, or anger; and they may feel detached or estranged from other people.[5] People with PTSD may avoid situations or people that remind them of the traumatic event, and they may have strong negative reactions to something as ordinary as a loud noise or accidental touch.[5] Critical care nurses spend most of their workday in the same environment that has caused their PTSD. In this situation, avoidance of the stress may necessitate a change in career. Recurrent exposure to these types of stressful events on a daily basis greatly increases the likelihood that PTSD will develop or be made worse. Now that PTSD has been generally defined and examined specifically related to critical care nurses, it is important to explore the signs and symptoms of this syndrome so that recognition and diagnosis occurs for at-risk nurses.

POSTTRAUMATIC STRESS DISORDER SIGNS AND SYMPTOMS

The signs and symptoms of PTSD are established by the American Psychological Association in collaboration with the National Institute of Mental Health. These diagnostic criteria are published in the *Diagnostic and Statistical Manual of Mental Disorders*, 5th edition.[5–7] For this article, the criteria are simplified.

Although specific symptoms can vary in severity, the symptoms of PTSD are divided into 4 categories (**Table 1**).[5–7]

Table 1
Four categories of posttraumatic stress disorder symptoms

Categories of Symptoms	Description of Categories
Intrusive thoughts	• Repeated involuntary memories, distressing dreams, or flashbacks of the traumatic event (vivid flashbacks in which individuals feel they are reliving the traumatic experience or visualizing the event)
Avoiding reminders of event	• Avoiding people, places, activities, objects, and situations that bring on distressing memories; resisting talking about what happened or how they feel about it
Negative thoughts or feelings	• Ongoing and distorted beliefs about oneself or others (eg, "I am bad," "No one can be trusted") • Ongoing fear, horror, anger, guilt, or shame • Less or lack of interest in activities previously enjoyed • Feeling detached or estranged from others
Arousal or reactive symptoms	• Irritable or angry outbursts • Reckless or self-destructive behavior • Easily startled • Difficulty with concentration or sleep

POSTTRAUMATIC STRESS DISORDER DIAGNOSIS CRITERIA

To be diagnosed with PTSD, an adult must have all the following for a duration of at least 1 month[5,7]:

- At least 1 reexperiencing symptom
- At least 1 avoidance symptom
- At least 2 arousal and reactivity symptoms
- At least 2 cognition and mood symptoms.

REEXPERIENCING SYMPTOMS

Reexperiencing symptoms may be flashbacks in which the individual is reliving the trauma repeatedly.[5,7] They may describe these symptoms as a physical indicator such as a racing heart, profuse sweating, the experience of bad dreams, and/or frightening thoughts. Reexperiencing symptoms may cause problems in a person's everyday routine. The symptoms can start from the person's thoughts and feelings. Words, objects, or situations that are reminders of the event can trigger reexperiencing symptoms.[5,7]

AVOIDANCE SYMPTOMS

Avoidance symptoms can cause individuals to stay away from places, events, or objects that are reminders of the traumatic experience.[5,7] Triggers may cause a person to change his or her routine. For example, after losing a patient with whom the critical care nurse developed close relationships with the patient and family, the nurse may try to avoid building relationships with future patients and families.[5,7]

Arousal and reactivity symptoms include[5,7]
- Being easily startled
- Feeling tense or on edge
- Having difficulty sleeping
- Having angry outbursts.

Arousal symptoms are usually constantly in the background. Rather than being triggered by things that remind one of the traumatic events, these behaviors and feelings may occur at any time. Arousal and reactivity symptoms can make the critical care nurse feel stressed and angry, and make it hard to perform daily tasks, such as sleeping and eating, Difficulty with concentration may also be a challenge.

Cognition and mood symptoms include[5,7]
- Trouble remembering key features of the traumatic event
- Negative thoughts about oneself or the world
- Distorted feelings such as guilt or blame
- Loss of interest in enjoyable activities.

Cognition and mood symptoms can begin or worsen after the traumatic event, or repeated exposure to said events by the critical care nurse. These symptoms can make the person feel alienated or detached from friends or family members.

PREVALENCE OF POSTTRAUMATIC STRESS DISORDER IN CRITICAL CARE NURSES

Nurses are at an increased risk for developing PTSD, especially nurses working on inpatient units.[8] Additionally, the risk of developing PTSD is multiplied in specialty areas of nursing, such as the critical care unit, emergency room, and oncology units.[9,10] PTSD occurs in critical care nurses at a rate of approximately 20% to 33%,[11] compared with 14% of general care nurses[8,12] and 8% to 10% of the general population of the United States.[9]

CONTRIBUTING FACTORS

The increased incidence of PTSD in critical care nurses is multifactorial. Nurses in intensive care units are repeatedly exposed to extremely stressful situations, including end-of-life care, cardiopulmonary resuscitation, and postmortem care.[4] Additionally, critical care nurses are more likely to see large open wounds, care for patients who are hemorrhaging, and witness patients dying.[9] Complicating an already difficult work environment, critical care nurses also report feeling that the work they do does not affect the outcome of the patient.[4] On average, 10% to 29% of all patients admitted to a critical care setting die during their hospitalization, often from intentional termination of life-support measures.[13]

Other factors that contribute to the incidence of PTSD include the age of the nurse, years in practice, and level of authority. There is conflicting information in the literature regarding the incidence of PTSD by the age of the nurse. In studies comparing critical care nurses to general care nurses, the incidence of PTSD decreased as the age of the nurse increased, and there was an inverse relationship between years of experience as a nurse and incidence of PTSD.[4,14] However, in contrast, a subsequent literature review by Mealer and Jones[9] (2013) demonstrated that the incidence of PTSD in critical care nurses is consistent regardless of the age of the nurse. It is noteworthy that nurses who assume the role of charge nurse are less likely to experience symptoms of PTSD than those who have never assumed the charge nurse role.[4,8] Nurses who use support systems and who have hobbies outside of work are also less likely to experience symptoms of job-related PTSD. Critical care nurses who reported poor or average coworker relationships were more likely to report symptoms of PTSD.[14]

CONSEQUENCES OF POSTTRAUMATIC STRESS DISORDER IN CRITICAL CARE NURSES

The imbalance of effort and result that comes from repeatedly caring for patients requiring high levels of care but are likely to have poor outcomes can result in other psychological symptoms in critical care nurses.[12] Critical care nurses who have PTSD are more likely to report irritability or agitation, and to experience muscle tension. These nurses also report having issues with sleeping, including nightmares, and describe having panic attacks related to their nursing experiences.[4] PTSD can contribute to impaired personal relationships and general decreased satisfaction with life.[8] A systematic review of dysfunctional responses in critical care nurses demonstrated that these nurses are more likely to report symptoms of anxiety and depression. The risk of anxiety and depression was also noted to be higher in nurses working the evening or night shift in the critical care unit.[4,12] Additionally, levels of increased anxiety and depression symptoms were not specific to the United States but were also found in critical care nurses in Greece, Nigeria, and France.[12] A single study in Turkey revealed the opposite; the investigators did not find a statistically significant difference in anxiety in critical care nurses compared with general care nursing staff. This study did, however, attribute increased stress to high levels of physical activity, which is common in critical care nurses.[12] It is important to note that differences in nursing responsibilities between nurses in the United States and in Turkey could be a factor in the levels of anxiety that the nurses report.

BURNOUT AND COMPASSION FATIGUE

Stress reactions as a consequence of the high acuity environment of critical care units can also lead to burnout and compassion fatigue in critical care nurses. Burnout is emotional exhaustion that leads nurses to feelings of being overwhelmed by their work. This can lead to the depersonalization of those receiving care and even a reduced perception of personal achievement. Critical care nurses who report having PTSD are more likely to report burnout,[8,10] with as many as 28% to 33% admitting to experiencing symptoms related to PTSD.[15] In nursing, death is a regular occurrence but a lack of nursing education related to death and how to effectively deal with it can lead to moral distress, which is often a precursor to burnout.[16] Other contributing factors that lead to burnout include heavy workloads, poor support systems, and bullying. Burnout can lead to increased fast-food consumption, infrequent exercise, and increased use of alcohol.[15] Additionally, there has been a positive correlation between medical errors and compromised patient safety when the nurse reports symptoms of burnout.[15] Absenteeism, or not coming in to work when scheduled, is also positively correlated with burnout.[17]

Compassion fatigue is defined as "physical or psychological distress in caregivers."[18] Loss of compassion can result from repeatedly caring for patients in disappointing situations, such as caring for patients in the critical care unit.[9] Nurses who suffer from compassion fatigue are less likely to be sympathetic to their patients' suffering,[18] and often report headaches, chest pain, mood swings, and irritability. Nurses who suffer from compassion fatigue are more likely to abuse alcohol and other substances.[15] Compassion fatigue can be a result of poor training, with a lack of appropriate nursing skills required to care for critically ill patients,[18] and is often the consequence of increased patient load due to nursing and ancillary staff shortages.[18] Compassion fatigue, like burnout, can lead to absenteeism and leaving the nursing profession.[18]

CONSEQUENCES OF NURSE POSTTRAUMATIC STRESS DISORDER FOR EMPLOYER

Nurses who develop PTSD and burnout syndrome work an average of 11.6 years less than nurses who do not report symptoms of PTSD and burnout.[15] The cost of nursing turnover to employers can be as high as $64,000 per nurse and can lead to decreased quality of patient care.[19] Critical care nurses report that stressful environments where they care for dying patients is a principal factor in their leaving the critical care unit.[19] Poor retention rates can also lead to increased stress for staff members who are left with a staffing shortage, not only in nurses but also in experienced nursing staff.[20] When more experienced nurses leave the critical care unit, nurses who have less experience are left to care for the patients are very ill and who need the highest level of expert care. The less experienced nurses face high levels of stress and diminished resources for assistance. Poor patient satisfaction scores have also been attributed to nurse burnout (a consequence of PTSD),[16] which can lead to a decrease in government funding for hospitals.

RESILIENCE

In looking at the consequences of PTSD in critical care nurses, many different detrimental issues have been covered and discussed. Attention is now shifted to what can be done to counteract and prevent the occurrence of PTSD in critical care nurses before it takes hold. In looking at previous theories and studies that have been advanced in this arena, the topic of resilience has shown the most promise in addressing this clinical issue. To discuss how resilience can play a role in combating PTSD in critical care nurses, it is important to first look at what resilience is and then examine factors that play a role in this possible solution. Resilience is a concept that refers to an individual's ability to bounce back or positively respond to adversity.[21] Resilience is also widely accepted as a psychological mechanism that can negate the effects of PTSD and is endorsed as among the most important factors for a beneficial recovery after experiencing trauma.[22] To some people, the ability to possess resilience comes naturally, whereas in others it does not. A lack of innate resilience does not mean that the trait cannot be learned. Psychological traits of resilience that can be taught and assimilated include engaging the support of colleagues and friends, learning and adopting effective coping skills, the use of humor, cognitive restructuring, and optimism.[23] It has been shown that critical care nurses with existing high levels of resilience are at a significantly lower risk of developing PTSD, depression, anxiety, and burnout syndrome.[24] In contrast, critical care nurses with symptoms of PTSD have reported problems with relationships, general life satisfaction, and overall functioning in all areas of their life.[8] Now that high resilience has been identified as a promising trait to combat PTSD development in critical care nurses, it is important to examine what contributes to the development of this positive psychological trait in nurses.

CONTRIBUTING FACTORS TO HIGH RESILIENCE

A review of literature shows there are 4 main domains that seem to play a pivotal role in supporting high resilience in critical care nurses. These domains are worldview, social network, cognitive flexibility, and self-care and balance. Although there is a wide breadth of knowledge on these topics as they relate to the development and sustainment of high resilience, they have been simplified for the purpose of this article.[25]

WORLDVIEW

Worldview refers to the individual nurse's fundamental understanding and belief in nursing care that serves as a framework through which a nurse can interpret the critical care work environment in relation to both positive and negative patient outcomes.[25] This foundation of worldview is primarily governed by a nurse's ethics, values, emotions, and previous experiences in the work environment. Highly resilient nurses are described as having a worldview that allows acceptance that death is a part of life and that patient outcomes cannot be controlled. This manner of acceptance does not diminish the highly resilient nurse's sense of hope for a patient's well-being but fosters a perspective that preserves psychological health adjustments by incorporating optimism and humor in the work environment.[25]

SOCIAL NETWORK

A social network is a structured organization of individuals that are connected formally and/or informally.[25] A nurse's social network provides communication, emotional support, and connectivity. The highly resilient nurse describes a positive social network, including close personal friendships, family relationships, and strong collegial relationships with fellow nurses and physicians whom they were able to draw on when needed. The unique aspect of this social network is that it offers a variety of relationships that are not entirely connected to the work environment.[25]

COGNITIVE FLEXIBILITY

Cognitive flexibility is a concept involving human behaviors and the ability to modify a response based on the contextual meaning of a situation.[25] Highly resilient nurses use emotional intelligence to guide decision-making and then incorporate methods such as critical reflection, optimism, and positive reframing to process the emotionally charged atmosphere of the critical care unit, as well as the indirect trauma caused by cumulative exposure in caring for critically ill patients. In addition to the stressors of the work environment, cognitive flexibility is also used to give meaning to previously experienced personal traumatic experiences that may have otherwise contributed to vicarious traumatization (being traumatized by hearing about another's trauma) and PTSD. In this manner, trauma is used more like a connecting gateway to humanity and is applied as a growing and/or learning experience. This translating of traumatic experiences into learning experiences has been conceptualized in the existing literature as posttraumatic growth.[25]

SELF-CARE AND BALANCE

Self-care and balance are the emotional, psychological, and physical mechanisms that are incorporated into daily living to maintain a balanced and healthy lifestyle.[25] Emotional health includes the recollection of positive experiences at work and the ability to leave stress at work. Psychological health includes rituals, coping mechanisms, and spirituality that are used in both the home and work environment. Physical health includes exercise, laughter, nutrition, and sleeping habits. The highly resilient nurse describes a life outside of work that includes many positive physical attributes, such as working out at the gym or running. They also are engaged in activities at work and home that highlight positive coping mechanisms, including engaging in prayer or spiritual rituals, using available social resources, and maintaining proper sleep patterns.[25]

So, in looking at the 4 main domains that have been shown to greatly contribute to high resilience in critical care nurses, it can be difficult to narrow down some of the more pertinent behaviors that have been proven effective. This step is important because it allows practicing nurses, nurse managers, and administrators to concentrate on which behaviors to select and foster among themselves and others. In a landmark study conducted by Mealer and colleagues,[25] highly resilient critical care nurses identified spirituality (92%) and social support (85%) as the most commonly used skills while working in the critical care environment. Other resilient characteristics used by the highly resilient critical care nurse included having a positive role model (54%), active coping skills (46%), and optimism (38%).[25] The identification of these pertinent behaviors will help arm administrative clinicians and organizational management with a blueprint that can then be used to create a framework by which they have the ability to identify and foster these behaviors in their critical care nursing staff.[25]

DISCUSSION

PTSD is a complex, and often debilitating, disorder that has far-reaching effects, including anxiety, depression, burnout, and compassion fatigue. Working as a nurse in a critical care unit can be physically and emotionally demanding. As a population, critical care nurses are at an increased risk of developing PTSD when compared with general care practice nurses. Companies that employ nurses are also affected due to increased rate of attrition, absenteeism, and general decreased quality in patient care in nurses who experience the consequences of PTSD. There is conflicting evidence related to which factors contribute to PTSD; however, increased resilience is the most promising factor to date in preventing PTSD.[25]

IMPLICATIONS FOR PRACTICE

Hospital administrators and nurse managers in critical care settings must be aware of the increased risk of PTSD in the critical care setting and the factors that contribute to the incidence of PTSD, as well as the implications of having staff with PTSD symptoms. One possible solution to consider is the assessment of staff mental health for those nurses who are hired to work in a critical care unit, followed by ongoing, consistent assessment while the nurse is employed in the critical care setting. Another opportunity for nurse managers and administration to decrease the risk of critical care nurses developing PTSD is to perform resilience testing on hire. The use of mental health assessment and resilience testing would alert the manager to nurses who might require closer observation for PTSD symptoms, and allow for early intervention, including resilience training, if symptoms are noted.

IMPLICATIONS FOR RESEARCH

Although PTSD has been investigated and has been demonstrated to be more common in critical care nurses than general care nurses and the general population, more research is needed regarding ways to identify nurses at risk for PTSD before their work is affected. Future research is also needed to investigate compassion fatigue and burnout related to PTSD, specifically patient outcomes after being cared for by nurses who report symptoms of PTSD with compassion fatigue or burnout. This research should focus on individual characteristics, as well as organizational characteristics, that contribute to PTSD in critical care nurses.

Resilience has been demonstrated to decrease adverse psychological outcomes for critical care nurses, including PTSD. For those nurses who demonstrate low levels of resilience during testing, resilience training has been demonstrated to decrease PTSD symptoms. This training should continue to be investigated, and research should focus specifically on the best ways to implement training and best practices for evaluation of the nurses who participate in the training.[25]

REFERENCES

1. Chan ZC, Tam WS, Lung MK, et al. A systematic literature review of nursing shortage and the intention to leave. J Nurs Manag 2013;21(4):605–13.
2. 2018 NSI national health care retention and RN staffing report. Available at: http://www.nsinursingsolutions.com/files/assets/library/retention-institute/nationalhealthcarernretentionreport2018.pdf. Accessed January 12, 2019.
3. Waldman JD, Kelly F, Arora S, et al. The shocking cost of turnover in healthcare. Health Care Manage Rev 2004;29(1):2–7.
4. Mealer ML, Shelton A, Berg B, et al. Increased prevalence of post-traumatic stress disorder symptoms in critical care nurses. Am J Respir Crit Care Med 2007;175(7):693–7.
5. American Psychiatric Association. What is posttraumatic stress disorder?. 2017. Available at: https://www.psychiatry.org/patients-families/ptsd/what-is-ptsd. Accessed January 14, 2019.
6. National Institute of Mental Health (NIMH). Post-traumatic disorder 2016. Available at: https://www.nimh.nih.gov/health/topics/post-traumatic-stress-disorder-ptsd/index.shtml. Accessed January 14, 2019.
7. American Psychiatric Association. Diagnostic and statistical manual of mental health disorders: DSM-5. 5th edition. Washington, DC: American Psychiatric Publishing; 2013.
8. Mealer M, Burnham E, Goode C, et al. The prevalence and impact of post-traumatic stress disorder and burnout syndrome in nurses. Depress Anxiety 2009;26:1118–26.
9. Mealer M, Jones J. Posttraumatic stress disorder in the nursing population: a concept analysis. Nurs Forum 2013;48(4):279–88.
10. Colville G, Smith J, Brierley J, et al. Coping with staff burnout and work-related posttraumatic stress in intensive care. Pediatr Crit Care Med 2017;18(7):267–73.
11. Cho G, Kang J. Type D personality and post-traumatic stress disorder symptoms among intensive care unit nurses; the mediating effect of resilience. PLoS One 2017;12(4):e0175067.
12. Karanikola M, Giannakopoulou M, Mpouzika M, et al. Dysfunctional psychological response among Intensive Care Unit nurses: a systematic review of the literature. Rev Esc Enferm USP 2015;49(5):847–57.
13. Noome M, Beneken Genaamd Kolmer DM, Van Leeuwen E, et al. The nursing role during end-of-life care in the intensive care unit related to the interaction between patient, family and professional: an integrative review. Scand J Caring Sci 2016; 30(4):645–61.
14. Von Rueden KT, Hinderer KA, McQuillan KA, et al. Secondary traumatic stress in trauma nurses: prevalence and exposure, coping, and personal/environmental characteristics. J Trauma Nurs 2010;17(4):191–200.
15. Azimi A, Hajiesmaeili M, Kangasniemi M, et al. Effects of stress on critical care nurses: a national cross-sectional study. J Intensive Care Med 2019. https://doi.org/10.1177/0885066617696853.
16. Brown S, Whichello R, Price S. The impact of resiliency on nurse burnout: an integrative literature review. Medsurg Nurs 2018;27(6):349–78.

17. Davey MM, Cummings G, Newburn-Cook CV, et al. Predictors of nurse absenteeism in hospitals: a systemic review. J Nurs Manag 2009;17(3):312–30.
18. Van Mol M, Kompanje E, Benoit D, et al. The prevalence of compassion fatigue and burnout among healthcare professionals in intensive care units: a systematic review. PLoS One 2015;10(8):e0136955.
19. Khan N, Jackson D, Stayt L, et al. Factors influencing nurses' intentions to leave adult critical care settings. Nurs Crit Care 2018;24(1):24–32.
20. Steinberg B, Klatt M, Duchemin A. Feasibility of a mindfulness-based intervention for surgical intensive care unit personnel. Am J Crit Care 2017;26(1):10–8.
21. Turner SB. The resilient nurse: an emerging concept. Nurs Lead 2014;12(6): 71–3, 90.
22. Earvolino-Ramirez M. Resilience: a concept analysis. Nurs Forum 2007;42:73–82.
23. Charney DS. Psychological mechanisms of resilience and vulnerability: implications for successful adaptation to extreme stress. Am J Psychiatry 2004;161(2): 195–216.
24. Mealer M, Jones J, Newman J, et al. The presence of resilience is associated with a healthier psychological profile in intensive care unit (ICU) nurses: results of a national survey. Int J Nurs Stud 2012;49(3):292–9.
25. Mealer M, Jones J, Moss M. A qualitative study of resilience and posttraumatic stress disorder in United States ICU nurses. Intensive Care Med 2012;38: 1445–51.

Burnout in Critical Care Nurses

Stacey G. Browning, DNP, MSN, RN

KEYWORDS

- Burnout • Critical care nurses • Intensive care unit • Maslach Burnout Inventory

KEY POINTS

- Burnout is a contested diagnosis with no official definition.
- Prevalence of burnout in critical care nurses varies widely because of the use of multiple evaluation tools and ambiguously structured components within the proposed construct of burnout.
- Perceived burnout has negative effects on individual nurses, patients and families, and health care organizations at large.

SCENARIO

The cardiovascular intensive care unit (CVICU) was short staffed, with only 6 nurses to manage 8 patients in a 27-bed CVICU. Three of those nurses were each assigned to 3 separate patients who had only arrived after change of shift from the operating suites after completion of their coronary artery bypass grafts. Two of the other nurses were each assigned 2 patients, and the last nurse was assigned 1 patient and 1 "hit-spot." Hit-spot was the term used to describe the room where the next admitted patient would be placed.

The hit-spot was quickly filled with a patient from the cardiac catheterization laboratory who had just undergone stent placement for an ST-elevated myocardial infarction (MI). In laymen's terms, the patient had experienced a heart attack requiring a device to be placed into an artery on the heart so that blood flow would be restored, and heart muscle saved. As a rule of thumb, all patients placed in CVICU were very sick. The MI patient was very sick. The patient was so sick that the reperfused heart stopped beating and the health care team (HCT) exhausted their limited human resources to help restart the patient's heart with cardiopulmonary resuscitation and medications.

In the meantime, 2 of the postoperative patients began spiraling downward, and soon the HCT was performing advanced cardiac life support on 2 patients. Two

Disclosure Statement: The author has nothing to disclose.
School of Nursing, College of Behavioral and Health Sciences, Middle Tennessee State University, PO Box 81, 1301 East Main, Murfreesboro, TN 37132, USA
E-mail address: Stacey.Browning@mtsu.edu

patients quickly became 3 patients, and then the rapid response call came loud and clear through the charge nurse telephone. The call was from a cardiac sister unit, and their patient at risk was likely one who had only recently left the care of the CVICU. The CVICU charge nurse's response was also loud and clear, "please call another rapid response team as we are unable to safely provide support due to managing three code situations with too few people."

When the shift was over and the dust had cleared, all 3 patients survived the night. The charge nurse rejoiced and breathed easier, until the unit manager appeared with bad news. She explained that the sister unit who had activated the rapid response team during the night reported to their manager that they had not been supported by the CVICU during their time of need. The charge nurse and other CVICU staff physically deflated at the news. They were already exhausted, both emotionally and physically, and all that they had worked to achieve was minimized by someone who had not been present and who had not valued their work ethic enough to ask about the scenario before assuming they had not been supportive of their peers. The CVICU staff walked away from that shift with a bitter taste in their mouths, feeling burned out.

BURNOUT SYNDROME

The case scenario above depicts a typical shift in any given critical care unit across the United States. Health care workers in critical care are under constant pressure, and like the providers in this scenario, often feel defeated, exhausted, and burned out. Burnout syndrome (burnout) was initially described by Herbert Freudenberger in 1974.[1–3] While maintaining his personal practice on the Upper East Side, Dr Freudenberger also worked pro bono with struggling, young drug addicts at his free clinic on Bowery, also known as New York City's Skid Row.[4] As a result of his continual work with, and dedication to, challenged populations, Dr Freudenberger began to feel irritable, exhausted, and unable to cope. It was then he used the term "burn-out" to infer a psychosocial disorder. Dr Freudenberger described burnout as feelings of fatigue and defeat secondary to overwhelming demands on vigor, vitality, or resources specifically as they relate to helping-professionals, such as the health care providers in the opening scenario.[5]

Christina Maslach and Susan E. Jackson continued to study the concept of burnout in the late 1970s and early 1980s. As a result of their research, Maslach and Jackson developed the widely used assessment tool titled the *Maslach Burnout Inventory* (MBI), which explicitly measured burnout frequency in helping professionals.[2,6–12] Maslach and Jackson postulated that burnout was a psychological syndrome that comprised 3 components, including emotional exhaustion (EE), depersonalization (D), and personal accomplishments (PA), which are defined in **Fig. 1**.[13,14] The MBI has been shown to be both reliable and valid as a tool to measure burnout in nurses, internationally.[15] However, the MBI has since been adapted from its original form and used to evaluate burnout in a variety of professions around the globe, which includes the Maslach Burnout Inventory–Human Services Survey for Medical Personnel (MBI-HHS [MP]).[1,14,15]

Evaluation Tools

The MBI was structured to evaluate a range of stress from zero to low levels of work-related stress, continuing through to low to high levels of burnout.[16] However, some have incorrectly operationalized the MBI to indicate the presence or absence of burnout as opposed to a continuum of work-related stress.[9,15–17] The MBI-HHS (MP) is a 22-item item survey consisting of 3 subscales, including EE, D, and PA.[18]

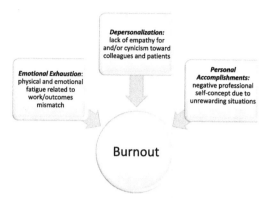

Fig. 1. Three components of burnout. (*Data from* Moss M, Good V, Gozal D, et al. A critical care societies collaborative statement: Burnout syndrome in critical care health-care professionals: A call for action. Am J Respir Crit Care Med. 2016;194(1):106–13.)

The EE dimension includes 9 items, while D contains 5 items, and PA consists of 8 items.[18] The survey is structured so that respondents score their job-related feelings in terms of frequency, as shown in **Table 1**.[18]

Although the MBI provides reliable, valid, and reproducible results, it was originally meant to evaluate burnout specifically in human service professionals, such as those working in health care.[19] Throughout the years, the MBI has been used to measure burnout in other professions and was eventually translated into separate MBI tools for various occupations. Other tools used to evaluate burnout include, but are not limited to, the Oldenburg Burnout Inventory, Physician Work-Life Study's Single Item, and the Copenhagen Burnout Inventory, which are all described in **Table 2**.[19]

Controversies

Although Dr Freudenberger recognized and continued to develop the concept of burnout beginning in 1974, there is still no official, scientific definition of burnout.[16,20] Burnout is not recognized as a mental disorder as evidenced by its lack of inclusion in the *Diagnostic and Statistical Manual of Mental Disorders*, which is maintained and developed by the American Psychiatric Association.[16,20] However, burnout is included and has been updated to reflect an "occupational phenomenon" (not a medical diagnosis) in the *International Classification of Diseases, 11th Revision (ICD-11)*, which is managed and updated by the World Health Organization (WHO).[16,20,21] The *ICD-11* is all-inclusive of conditions that influence the holistic/medical well-being of the global society.[21] The *ICD-11* aims to streamline medical vocabulary and statistics and is

Table 1
Maslach Burnout Inventory–Human Services Survey for Medical Personnel example

	Never	A Few Times a Year or Less	Once a Month or Less	A Few Times a Month	Once a Week	A Few Times a Week	Every Day
1. "I feel emotionally drained from my work."							

Reproduction by special permission of the Publisher, Mind Garden, Inc., www.mindgarden.com from the Maslach Burnout Inventory Human Services Survey by Christina Maslach & Susan E. Jackson. Copyright © 1981 by Christina Maslach & Susan E. Jackson. Further Reproduction is prohibited without the Publisher's written consent.

Table 2
Tools to evaluate the presence of burnout

Tool	Date	Birthplace	Purpose	Format	Validated Applications
1. Maslach Burnout Inventory–Human Services for Medical Personnel	1981	United States	Measures burnout in human services professionals[19]	22-item survey with 3 areas: EE, DP, & low sense of PA[19]	*Patients:* adults *Population:* helping professionals *Setting:* helping professions[19]
2. Physician Work-Life Study's Single Item	2000	United States	Measures burnout in any occupational group[19]	Single item. Respondents rate overall burnout from 1 (no burnout) to 5 (complete burnout)[19]	*Patients:* adults *Population:* physicians *Setting:* any health care setting[19]
3. Copenhagen Burnout Inventory	2005	Denmark	Measures burnout in any occupational group[19]	19-Item survey covering 3 areas: personal, work, and client related[19]	*Patients:* adults *Population:* any occupational group *Setting:* any[19]
4. Oldenburg Burnout Inventory	2002	Germany	Measures burnout in any occupational group[19]	16-Item survey covering 2 areas: exhaustion and work disengagement[19]	*Patients:* adults *Population:* any occupational group *Setting:* any[19]

Data from National Academy of Sciences. Validated instruments to assess work-related dimensions of well-being. Available at: https://nam.edu/valid-reliable-survey-instruments-measure-burnout-well-work-related-dimensions/. Accessed February 8, 2019.

used globally to allocate health care and financial resources where needed.[21] In the United States, the *ICD-11* is used to guide health care insurance billing, which may add complexity for providers and patients.[21] Although using a common language lends itself to tracking global health issues, the *ICD* has traditionally been cumbersome and difficult to use, which has previously contributed to skewed data.[21] The *ICD-11* revision process included efforts to simplify codes in the hope of making it easier for care providers to use.[21]

Scientists, researchers, and educators continue to disagree as to the legitimacy of the concept of burnout.[15,16,20] Many professionals chide there are too many overlapping symptoms between burnout and other previously established mental disorders, such as depression, as shown in **Table 3**.[15,16,20] However, professionals who support burnout as a unique process posit the largest difference as having to do with the relativity of burnout symptoms to work, thereby making it the occupational phenomenon as defined by the WHO.[2–14,16–22] In other words, burnout is associated with work, whereas depression is not, although burnout may increase the risk of developing depression and posttraumatic stress disorder.[10,13,14,22,23]

RISK FACTORS

The Critical Care Societies Collaborative (CCSC) describes 4 categories of risk factors associated with burnout, as shown in **Fig. 2**.[14] The CCSC consists of 4 professional and scientific societies of the United States, including the American Association of Critical-Care Nurses, the American College of Chest Physicians, the American Thoracic Society, and the Society of Critical Care Medicine.[14] In consideration of the introductory scenario, the CVICU staff experienced risks associated with burnout in 3 of the 4 CCSC categories, including organizational factors, exposure to end-of-life issues, and poor quality of working relationships. Individually, the charge nurse was self-critical of the way she had managed the shift and wondered what she could or should have done differently.

In addition to the components listed in **Fig. 2**, there are other individual and organizational characteristics and traits that contribute to the development of burnout, including working in critical care areas where increased patient morbidity and mortality lend themselves to ethical dilemmas, and mentally and physically demanding daily practices.[2,9,10,12–14,18,22–24] Those working in academic hospitals, and individuals who possess such traits as neuroticism, self-deprecation, extraversion, meticulousness, and poor coping strategies are at risk for burnout.[7,14,23] Perceived organizational values and justice conflicts both contribute to increased risk of burnout, as does poor or no social support from colleagues and supervisors.[23,24] However, other studies have indicated burnout as a contagious phenomenon existing especially among teams of the same area or unit, such as the HCT in the case scenario.[14,25] It has also been suggested that transactional leadership contributes to staff burnout as

Table 3 Symptoms associated with burnout and depression		
Shared Symptoms	**Depression**	**Burnout**
Extreme exhaustion	Hopelessness	Lack of empathy
Inability to feel happy	Low self-esteem	Being unprofessional
Reduced performance	Suicidal tendencies	Feeling insufficient at work

Data from Informed Health. What is burnout? Available at: https://www.informedhealth.org/what-is-burnout.2125.en.html?part=symptome-5i. Accessed July 26, 2019.

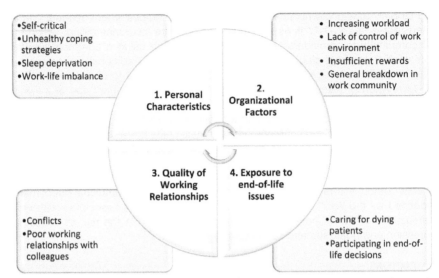

- Self-critical
- Unhealthy coping strategies
- Sleep deprivation
- Work-life imbalance

1. Personal Characteristics

2. Organizational Factors

- Increasing workload
- Lack of control of work environment
- Insufficient rewards
- General breakdown in work community

3. Quality of Working Relationships

4. Exposure to end-of-life issues

- Conflicts
- Poor working relationships with colleagues

- Caring for dying patients
- Participating in end-of-life decisions

Fig. 2. Risk categories associated with burnout. (*Data from* Moss M, Good V, Gozal D, et al. A critical care societies collaborative statement: Burnout syndrome in critical care health-care professionals: A call for action. Am J Respir Crit Care Med. 2016;194(1):106–13.)

well as high nurse-to-patient staffing ratios.[24] Along with critical care staff, studies have indicated those working in emergency and oncologic areas also experience a higher incidence of burnout.[10,12,18,24–26]

Prevalence

The prevalence of burnout varies widely across studies in part because of disparities in the tools used to measure burnout as well as scoring methods, multiple professional categories and occupations studied, cross-cultural variances, and varied international, organizational, and unit-based workloads and resources.[9,10,12,14–18,25–27] Variation in scoring methods contributes to the wide range of burnout prevalence and intensity, which varies from 0% to 80% in critical care nurses.[8–10,14] International variation in the prevalence of burnout may occur in relation to cultural differences, which influence psychosocial factors.[15,17,26,27]

Just as international variation contributes to cultural difference, so too do organizational, and even unit-level, variations, which may be influenced by shared morals, values, beliefs, and mismatched resources.[15,17,23] It has also been postulated that areas with longer lengths of stay have less incidence of burnout among staff when compared with units with shorter lengths of stay.[15] The rationale for increasing rates of burnout among those working in units with shorter lengths of stay stems from the frequency and speed at which patients are admitted, treated, and discharged, which all increase the workload of staff.[15]

CONSEQUENCES OF BURNOUT

The consequences of burnout negatively affect individual, organizational, and unit-level outcomes. When individuals experience burnout and do not recognize symptoms or take corrective action, the negative personal effects may include both physical and emotional manifestations. High stress may contribute to lethargy, which may be worsened by difficulty sleeping.[23,24] Feelings of emotional instability and cynicism contribute to apathy among nurses, who feel as though they can no longer support the psychological needs of their patients.[6,10,23,24] Nurses experiencing burnout often have, or develop, unhealthy coping techniques, such as emotion-focused or defensive coping mechanisms.[23,24] Emotion-focused coping describes alcohol, substance, or eating disorders, whereas defensive coping mechanisms include denial, isolation, and the use of humor to detract from the actual problem.[23,24] All the previously mentioned symptoms are likely to make nurses more susceptible to illnesses as well as decrease job satisfaction.[7,23,24,27] Physical illnesses commonly associated with burnout include cardiovascular disease, hypertension, and diabetes mellitus type 2.[23]

Many researchers posit the organizational and unit-level repercussions of burnout to include decreased quality of care, poor communication with patients and families, increased staff turnover, absenteeism, and low morale.[6,7,10–12,14,22] Other organizational costs incurred as a result of staff burnout include decreased patient satisfaction, increased patient and family distrust, and increased medical errors.[7,9–12,14,22] Increased health care costs are associated with increased staff turnover as well as increased rates of 30-day patient morbidity and mortality, which have both been linked to higher rates of staff burnout.[14]

Professional Anecdote

Bedside nursing is one of the most rewarding professional roles I have ever performed. It was also one of the most challenging roles because deficient communication and resources contributed to my own perceived poor quality of care. The example presented in the opening scenario is not in isolation, because I experienced similar situations, which ultimately contributed to a precipitous decline in team morale. I have worn many hats as a registered nurse, including critical care nurse, progressive care nurse, patient flow nurse, nurse leader, and nurse educator. Participating in excellently designed and well-executed HCT rounds had a tremendously positive impact on streamlining provider communication and patient care, which, research suggests, contributes to decreased levels of perceived burnout.[10,17] In those areas that have implemented and continued developing successful HCT rounds, it has been my perception that patients and families are placed as the central component of care with nurses as their personal advocates for developing and delivering appropriate and effective care plans.

It has also been my experience in areas without structured HCT rounds that I was often left wondering what the plan of care will be for the day in addition to receiving multiple (and conflicting) plans of care from various medical teams who may or may not speak directly to each other, or to me, the primary nurse. My experiences are not in isolation, and likely most nurses practicing bedside care can provide similar anecdotes. Although I was unaware of the concept of burnout at the time, I now look back on those daily bedside nurse challenges and understand they motivated me to seek advanced nursing degrees and leadership roles so that I could positively contribute to a culture of team and encourage bedside nurses to thrive at their fullest potential.

THERAPEUTIC INTERVENTIONS

Even though burnout is a hypothetical diagnosis in the United States, it has continued to be studied and developed, and interventions have been operationalized internationally.[17] Preventative measures, such as mindfulness training and communication techniques, especially in relation to end-of-life care, have reduced burnout by as much as

60% in some studies.[17] The addition of HCT rounding, ethics committees, robust palliative care teams, open visitation for families, stress debriefing, and counselors as needed for staff has contributed to reducing the incidence of burnout.[10,17] In addition, studies have shown a positive correlation between therapeutic interventions, such as research groups, coping, cognitive and stress-management training, team-building, and social support, and decreased levels of burnout.[10,17] Staff who received positive feedback reported decreased levels of burnout.[10,17] In the introductory CVICU scenario, the HCT should have received positive feedback as well as the opportunity for stress debriefing after an emotionally charged and physically demanding shift.

Team Strategies and Tools to Enhance Performance and Patient Safety (TeamSTEPPS) is a training tool developed by the Department of Defense's Patient Safety Program in partnership with the Agency for Healthcare Research and Quality to assist health care workers advance communication, with the goal of improving patient safety and quality of care.[22,28] It is a systematic approach to reducing unnecessary steps or traits. TeamSTEPPS reduces organizational and personal traits that contribute to poor communication and teamwork. Conversely, it promotes positive communication techniques and teamwork. Research has shown improved intensive care unit (ICU) and hospital lengths of stay as well as reduced mortalities and overall cost of care with the team model.[29,30] HCT rounding and the addition of critical care pharmacists and respiratory therapists can improve total patient care in the team model.[29,30] However, studies also outline the barriers to implementing and developing the team model, which include shortages of all ICU health care providers, including nurses who should not have a greater patient ratio than 1:2 in the critical care setting.[29,30]

Mindfulness is a technique being used to prevent and/or reduce burnout in critical care HCTs.[31] Mindfulness is the practice of being present and relaxed in the moment, while accepting what is happening around us, without feelings of exasperation.[31] Mindfulness includes short pauses throughout the day to meditate and may be combined with yoga or sports. When operationalized as part of critical care nursing education and training, nurses reported decreased levels of perceived stress, less likelihood of experiencing varying degrees of burnout, more focused work, and improved overall well-being.[30–33]

SUMMARY

Burnout syndrome is a contested diagnosis that is not recognized in the United States, although the concept of burnout has been studied and modified in health care professionals since its recognition as a unique psychological state of being by Dr Freudenberger in 1974. Critical care registered nurses work in a challenging environment that invokes feelings of stress, lack of support, emotional instability, loss of physical and mental well-being, and increased staff turnover. In turn, the provision of patient care suffers, and patients and families experience distrust of staff, poor communication, decreased quality of care and satisfaction, and ultimately, increased patient morbidity and mortality. All the previously mentioned challenges contribute to increasing the already exorbitant financial cost of care to both health care organizations and the general public.

Because burnout is not a recognized diagnosis in the United States, there is conflict regarding the legitimacy of burnout and whether those nurses who experience burnout are really suffering from other mental disorders, such as depression. Without complete support and agreement of the scientific and medical communities, research will continue to reflect a concept in limbo without advancements as to prevalence, prevention and treatment, and the long-term efficacy of such therapeutic interventions to reduce burnout among critical care nurses. Lack of consensus regarding burnout discourages accurate data reflective of a true crisis among critical care nurses and makes prevention and treatment outcomes difficult to measure. Moving forward, researchers and medical professionals should work together to determine the validity of the concept of burnout.[34]

REFERENCES

1. Montero-Marin J, Garcia-Campayo J, Mosquera Mera D, et al. A new definition of burnout syndrome based on Farber's proposal. J Occup Med Toxicol 2009;4(31). https://doi.org/10.1186/1745-6673-4-31.
2. Pastores S. Burnout syndrome in ICU caregivers. CHEST 2016;150(1):1–2.
3. Freudenberger H. Staff burn-out. J Soc Issues 1974;30(1):159–65.
4. King N. When a psychologist succumbed to stress, he coined the term 'burnout'. National Public Radio, Inc; 2016. Available at: https://www.npr.org/2016/12/08/504864961/when-a-psychologist-succumbed-to-stress-he-coined-the-term-burn out. Accessed January 26, 2019.
5. Freudenberger HJ. The staff burn-out syndrome in alternative institutions. Psychotherapy: Theory, Research & Practice 1975;12(1):73–82.
6. Maslach C, Jackson SE. The measurement of experienced burnout. J Occup Behav 1981;2:99–113.
7. Canadas-De la Fuente G, Vargas C, San Luis C, et al. Risk factors and prevalence of burnout syndrome in the nursing profession. Int J Nurs Stud 2014; 52(2015):240–9.
8. Mealer M. Burnout syndrome in the intensive care unit: future directions for research. Ann Am Thorac Soc 2015;13(7):997–8.
9. Fumis R, Amarante G, Nascimento A, et al. Moral distress and its contribution to the development of burnout syndrome among critical care providers. Ann Intensive Care 2017;7(71):1–8.
10. Poncet M, Toullic P, Papazian L, et al. Burnout syndrome in critical care nursing staff. Am J Respir Crit Care Med 2007;175:698–704.
11. Laschinger H, Fida R. New nurses burnout and workplace wellbeing: the influence of authentic leadership and psychological capital. Burn Res 2014;1: 19–28.
12. Elshaer N, Moustafa M, Aiad M, et al. Job stress and burnout syndrome among critical care healthcare workers. Alexandria Journal of Medicine 2017;54:273–7.
13. Mealer M, Moss M, Good V, et al. What is burnout syndrome (BOS)? Am J Respir Crit Care Med 2016;194(1):1–2.
14. Moss M, Good V, Gozal D, et al. A Critical Care Societies Collaborative Statement: burnout syndrome in critical care health-care professionals: a call for action. Am J Respir Crit Care Med 2016;194(1):106–13.
15. Poghosyan L, Aiken L, Sloane D. Corrigendum to "Factor structure of the Maslach burnout inventory: an analysis of data from large scale cross-sectional surveys of nurses from eight countries". Int J Nurs Stud 2014;51(10):1416–7.
16. Heinemann L, Heinemann T. Burnout research: emergence and scientific investigation of a contested diagnosis. Sage Open 2017;7(1):1–12.
17. van Mol M, Kompanje E, Benoit D, et al. The prevalence of compassion fatigue and burnout among healthcare professionals in intensive care units: a systematic review. PLoS One 2015;10(8):1–22.

18. Validated instruments to assess work-related dimensions of well-being. National Academy of Sciences; 2019. Available at: https://nam.edu/valid-reliable-survey-instruments-measure-burnout-well-work-related-dimensions/. Accessed February 8, 2019.
19. MBI: Human Services Survey for Medical Personnel. Mind Garden; 2019. Available at: https://www.mindgarden.com/315-mbi-human-services-survey-medical-personnel. Accessed February 17, 2019.
20. Bianchi R, Schonfeld I, Laurent E. Is it time to consider "burnout syndrome" a distinct illness? Front Public Health 2015;3(158):1–3.
21. Depression: what is burnout? Informed health online. Available at: https://www.ncbi.nlm.nih.gov/books/NBK279286/. Accessed January 27, 2019.
22. van Bogaert P, Timmermans O, Mace Weeks S, et al. Nursing unit teams matter: impact of unit-level nurse practice environment, nurse work characteristics, and burnout on nurse reported job outcomes, and quality of care, and patient adverse events–a cross-sectional survey. Int J Nurs Stud 2014;51:1123–34.
23. Job burnout: how to spot it and take action. Mayo Clinic; 2018. Available at: https://www.mayoclinic.org/healthy-lifestyle/adult-health/in-depth/burnout/art-20046642. Accessed January 27, 2019.
24. Bria M, Baban A, Dumitrascu D. Systematic review of burnout risk factors among European healthcare professionals. Cogn Brain Behav 2012;10(3):423–52.
25. Bakker A, Le Blanc P, Schaufeli Q. Burnout contagion among intensive care nurses. J Adv Nurs 2005;51(3):276–87.
26. Rushton C, Batcheller J, Schroeder K, et al. Burnout and resilience among nurses practicing in high-intensity settings. Am J Crit Care 2015;24(5):412–20.
27. Vargas C, Canadas G, Aguayo R, et al. Which occupational risk factors are associated with burnout in nursing? A meta-analytic study. Int J Clin Health Psychol 2014;14(1):28–38.
28. About TeamSTEPPS. Agency for Healthcare Research and Quality; 2017. Available at: https://www.ahrq.gov/teamstepps/about-teamstepps/index.html. Accessed February 17, 2019.
29. Durbin CG Jr. Team model: advocating for the optimal method of care delivery in the intensive care unit. Crit Care Med 2006;34(3 Suppl):S12–7.
30. Eppich WJ, Brannen M, Hunt EA. Team training: implications for emergency and critical care pediatrics. Curr Opin Pediatr 2008;20(3):255–60.
31. Lan H, Subramanian P, Rahmat N, et al. The effects of mindfulness training program on reducing stress and promoting well-being among nurses in critical care units [online]. Aust J Adv Nurs 2014;31(3):22–31. Available at: https://search.informit.com.au/documentSummary;dn=285671898965330;res=IELAPA.
32. Gauthier T, Meyer R, Grefe D, et al. An on-the-job mindfulness-based intervention for pediatric ICU nurses: a pilot. J Pediatr Nurs 2014;30(2):402–9.
33. Said Z, Kheng GL. A review on mindfulness and nursing stress among nurses. Analitika 2018;10(1):31–45.
34. Harvey EJ. Burnout should not be a silent epidemic. Can J Surg 2019;62(1):4–5.

Management Strategies in the Intensive Care Unit to Improve Psychosocial Outcomes

Lynn C. Parsons, PhD, MSN, RN, NEA-BC[a],[*],
Michele A. Walters, DNP, APRN, FNP-BC[b],[1]

KEYWORDS

- Intensive care • Patient and family needs • Post-ICU syndrome • Technologies
- Communication • Psychological distress • ICU diaries • ICU delirium

KEY POINTS

- Nurses practicing in intensive care units across the country have positively affected psychosocial metrics for delivering holistic care; helped patients and their families cope with injury, illness, and death; practiced nonpharmacologic interventions; helped patients return to their home environments and community; provided education to the patient and their family; delivered quality care; and served as strong patient advocates.
- The Model of Professional Nursing Practice provides guidance to committed critical care nurses in the provision of safe care delivery and contributing to quality patient outcomes based on current evidence-based practices.
- Early rehabilitation reduces the impact of postintensive care syndrome for survivors of critical illness.

INTRODUCTION

Year after year, nurses earn the distinction of being the most honest and ethical among several different professionals.[1,2] Nurses have received this accolade every year since 1999, with the exception of 2001 when firefighters scored at the top as a result of the 9/11 terrorist attack in New York City. In this society, patients realize positive psychosocial outcomes in the most critical care environments through care received in intensive care units (ICUs) across the country. The Model for Professional Nursing Regulation provides practice guidance for ICU nurses that can lead to positive

Disclosure Statement: The authors have nothing to disclose.
[a] Center for Health, Education and Research, Morehead State University, 316 West Second Street, Suite 201P, Morehead, KY 40351, USA; [b] St. Claire Family Medicine Express, Morehead State University, 316 West Second Street, CHER 201F, Morehead, KY 40351, USA
[1] Present address: 306 Meadow Lane, Morehead, KY 40351.
[*] Corresponding author. 817 Greenfield Trail, Mount Sterling, KY 40353.
E-mail address: l.parsons@moreheadstate.edu

psychosocial outcomes associated with critical care nurse practice. This article focuses on psychosocial outcomes associated with patients, their families, and nurses who practice on ICUs across the United States.

INTENSIVE CARE NURSING

Nurses practicing in ICUs must have strong clinical skills to care for persons with life-threatening injuries and illnesses. They must have a systematic method to organize care, be good multitaskers, and have stellar critical thinking and diagnostic reasoning skills.[3] Hamstra[4] (2018), an ICU nurse described nurses practicing in ICUs as, "Meticulous, organized, planners, loves detailed level of care, and they can simultaneously orchestrate 10 pumps, 6 drips, 4 beeps, and 1 crashing patient without blinking an eye."

There are many different specialty ICUs across the country: pediatric, cardiac, medical, surgical, cardiovascular, neurologic, and so forth. These units are staffed with several different health professionals. Intensive care nursing evolved as a specialty in the 1970s. Registered nurses (RNs) practicing in ICUs are augmented with advanced practice RNs (APRNs), mainly acute care nurse practitioners, and clinical nurse specialists.[5] These professionals help the team in collaborative patient care management, provide for patient and family education, and help deliver holistic care.[6]

MAJOR PSYCHOSOCIAL SUPPORTS PROVIDED BY NURSES IN THE INTENSIVE CARE UNIT

Nurses contribute every day to strategies that help patients and their families adjust and cope with major illnesses. Major psychosocial outcomes are realized through thoughtful practice provided by RNs and APRNs, including clinical nurse specialists, in ICUs across the country. **Box 1** presents positive psychosocial outcomes that nurses contribute to on a daily basis in multiple specialty ICUs.[5]

Holistic Approach

Adverse psychosocial consequences in ICUs can be averted or minimized if a holistic approach to patient care and interactions with families is practiced.[6] There are several techniques that the critical care nurse can use to demonstrate caring and delivery of a holistic approach to patient and family care:

- Speak directly to the patient and/or their family by using their name.
- Smile and use good eye contact.

Box 1
Psychosocial outcomes supported by nurses

- Holistic care
- Coping with illness, injury, or death
- Nonpharmacological interventions
- Reintegration into community
- Knowledge
- Quality care
- Advocacy

- When entering the room, provide a warm greeting, "Good morning, Mr Campbell."
- Ask how the patient is doing, showing genuine care and concern.
- Provide for privacy for intrusive procedures, toileting, and so forth.
- Use nonpharmacological interventions, such as soft music, repositioning, or adjusting pillows, to promote comfort.
- Help the patient and/or family understand simple or complex health care procedures before initiating them, to minimize anxiety.
- Be cognizant of nonverbal communications.
- Ask the patient if they need a question answered or a procedure explained.
- Make rounds with the medical team to hear what is being said to the patient.
- Act as a liaison between the patient or family and the medical team. Go into the room after to see if the patient understood what was said by the medical team. Reinforce that all questions that the patient and/or family have are important and that nothing is too basic to ask.
- Personalize interactions as much as possible: shake a family member's hand or touch the arm of the patient and/or family member.[6]

Nurses practicing in critical care make decisions and recommendations and engage in ethical practice, thus bolstering their commitment to patients and their families. Nurse practice consistent with the American Nurses Association (ANA) Code of Ethics facilitates this assurance to the public. The ANA Code of Ethics acknowledges the role of critical care nurses in treating patients and their families with dignity, and respecting them and their religious, spiritual, and cultural beliefs while maintaining privacy and confidentiality.[7]

The advanced technologies associated with care delivery in ICUs must be balanced by nurses through personalized care and compassion. Communication of pertinent information to the family and reassuring them that they will be notified for any change in their loved one's condition helps to provide comprehensive, holistic care. Environments in ICUs can be perceived by patients and families as sterile, noisy and impersonal. Early research completed by Heyland and colleagues[8] cites that families report the need to be in close proximity to their family member and their need for comfort. Comfort needs can be met by having a private family room area with a telephone, pillows, and blankets; access to refreshments; and providing a television and computer access. These types of activities contribute to taking care of the whole patient.[6]

Coping with Illness, Injury, and Death

Providing patients and their families with accurate information helps establish trust and a way to cope with uncomfortable treatment plans, such as dressing changes for a burn patient, or an activity or exercise regimen for an orthopedic patient. Helping a patient or family member deal with a terminal illness and eventual patient death openly and honestly can facilitate end-of-life care and decision-making. Involvement with child care arrangements and financial concerns, such as the monthly mortgage payment, facilitates a dying patient's need to care for family while simultaneously providing reassurance to the family being left behind.[9]

Early evidence reported by Leske[9] supports that communicating pertinent information to the family, encouraging them to be near their loved one, providing assurances, providing comfort measures to the family as much as possible within an ICU setting, and having support available helps people cope with critical illnesses. Consultations with different members of the health care team can provide needed assistance. For example, consulting with a social worker to provide health insurance information;

social or familial concerns, such as child care provision; and personal financial information can ease the mind of a dying person while providing the family with needed information.

Nonpharmacological Coping Interventions

Chaing and colleagues[10] conducted a study supporting the use of a Brief Cognitive-Behavior Psycho-Education (B-CBE) program for managing stress and anxiety in main family caregivers of patients in the ICU. The main caregiver was provided 1-on-1 instruction regarding physiologic, emotional, behavioral, and cognitive response of stress and anxiety using Beck's Cognitive Behavioral approach. During a 2-hour session that used mini-talks, exercises, and active discussion, the main family caregiver was provided information on stress awareness, cognitive recognition, and intervention with breathing and relaxation exercises. Chaing and colleagues[10] (2016) concluded that the use of brief interventions aimed to provide psychological education of cognitive behavioral management strategies demonstrated that the main family caregivers were more in control of their cognitive processes and were able to grieve in a less destructive manner when loss occurred than those in the control group. The B-CBE group reported higher information satisfaction scores than the control group after the program. Larger sample studies implementing a B-CBE program by critical care nurses needs to be conducted to explore the impact of a B-CBE program.[10]

Psychological distress is not only encountered by the main family caregivers but also by the patient. Postintensive care syndrome (PICS) is often experienced by survivors of critical illness who display new or worsening impairments of physical, cognitive, and/or mental health.[11] Early rehabilitation in the ICU may reduce complications associated with PICS. Evidence from a Johns Hopkins Hospital quality improvement project supports the dedication of a full-time physical therapist and occupational therapist to the ICU to improve physical function among mechanically ventilated patients, which in turn improves their psychological functioning.[11] Protocols and order sets have been found to improve the effectiveness of implementing an early rehabilitation program. The benefits for patients participating in early rehabilitation in the ICU include improved muscle strength, physical function, and quality of life.[11]

Additional strategies to decrease the occurrence of PICS is through the use of ICU diaries by the nurse and family. Garrouste-Orgeas and colleagues[12] demonstrated that an ICU diary significantly reduced symptoms related to posttraumatic stress in relatives and surviving patients 12 months after ICU discharge. Clinical research supports the use of these simple and inexpensive ICU diaries to reduce post-ICU mental health complications. An international ICU diary network is an online resource to aid in implementation of diaries in an ICU setting.[13]

Experiences while in the ICU may be long-lasting and have adverse effects on patients' cognitive-affective functioning.[14] Preventing long-lasting effects and efforts to improve overall psychological wellbeing should be incorporated into patient care. Interventions need to be considered to assess, prevent, and manage ICU delirium. ICU delirium is a predictor of increased mortality and prolonged hospitalization, and is associated with long-term cognitive impairment.[15]

ICU delirium should be monitored in all patients but those with increased risk should be identified. Kotfits and colleagues[15] outline risk factors for ICU delirium (**Table 1**).

Vanderbilt University developed an easy-to-remember mnemonic for quick analysis of delirium (**Box 2**). Using this mnemonic, ICU nurses will be able to identify patients on admission by recognizing predisposing and precipitating factors. Prodeliric drugs should be removed from the patient's plan of care.[15]

Table 1		
Risk factors for intensive care unit delirium		
Predisposing Factors		
Older age		
Frailty		
History of cognitive disorders		
Alcohol and/or drug abuse		
Severity of the underlying disease		
Precipitating Factors		
Precipitating Disorders		**Precipitating Drugs**
Metabolic disorders		Benzodiazepines
Ion disorders		Opioids (morphine)
Hypotension		Anticholinergic drugs
Sepsis		Steroids
Inadequate pain management		Deep sedation
Mechanical ventilation		
Sleep disorders		
Complicated surgery (abdominal cavity, cardiac surgery, femoral neck fracture)		

Adapted from Kotfits K, Marra A, Ely EW. ICU delirium: a diagnostic and therapeutic challenge in the intensive care unit. Republished with permission from: Anaesthesiology Intensive Therapy, 2018; 50: 2, 128–140.

Nonpharmacological interventions, such as providing access to hearing aids, glasses, orientation to time and situation, and decreased environmental noise, should be implemented before considerations of pharmacologic agents to control symptoms of delirium.[15]

Box 2
Prevention and early intervention for intensive care unit delirium
Stop
Remove all precipitating drugs or consider withdrawal syndromes:
Benzodiazepines
Anticholinergic drugs (metoclopramide, histamine-blockers, promethazine, diphenhydramine)
Steroids
THINK (mnemonic)
Toxins: congestive heart failure, shock, dehydration, delirium-inducing drugs, new failure of the liver or kidneys
Hypoxemia
Infections or sepsis, inflammation, immobilization
Nonpharmacological interventions: early mobility or early exercises, hearing aids, glasses, time or space orientation, sleep hygiene, music, noise control
K^+ (potassium ion) disturbances and disturbances of other electrolytes, metabolic disturbances
Finally, medicate
Classical antipsychotic drugs (eg, haloperidol)
Atypical antipsychotic drugs (eg, quetiapine)
Alfa-2 agonists (eg, dexmedetomidine, clonidine)

From Kotfits K, Marra A, Ely EW. ICU delirium: a diagnostic and therapeutic challenge in the intensive care unit. Republished with permission from: Anaesthesiology Intensive Therapy, 2018; 50: 2, 128–140.

Reintegration into the Community

After a critical illness it is important to help the patient and family return to the community and their home setting. Adaptations may have to be made within the home environment to ensure safety. A referral to a home health agency may be needed, at least initially, to assist the patient in acclimating in returning to their home and functioning as independently as possible. The patient's independence can be eased through use of adaptive equipment and simple rearrangement of furniture. The patient may have to adapt and cope with temporary placement in a long-term care center to receive needed therapy before they can independently complete self-care in their home.[8]

Nurses contribute to patient's self-care through patient education in the ICU settings. They teach family members treatment techniques, such as dressing changes and medication administration, before discharge, to facilitate patient independence and autonomy after discharge. The role of educating patients and their families is much more challenging today due to reduced patient length of stay in the ICU and the hospital compared with the past. Nurses have a duty to educate the patient, which is supported by the ANA Code of Ethics.[7]

Quality Care Delivery

Nurses provide best care when they are current in practice and are knowledgeable in best evidence-based practices. Quality care delivery enhances patient safety and promotes positive patient outcomes.[3] Nurses contribute to quality care delivery though many different mechanisms (**Table 2**).

Advocacy

The role of the critical care nurse as a patient advocate is especially important because nurses often care for individuals who cannot speak for themselves.[16] This includes persons who are mentally impaired, children, unconscious, uneducated, or intimidated by their provider or the health system.[17–19] The ANA Code of Ethics clearly articulates that the nurse has a professional responsibility to protect the rights of patients and act as a patient advocate.[20]

The nurse provides a link between the patient and the health system to help patients and families with making informed decisions.[21] The ICU nurse advocates for the best

Table 2	
Intensive care unit nurses' contributions to quality care	
Event	**Example**
Active participation in unit task forces and committees	Published patient education materials for patient or families on a variety of pertinent topics
Places research evidence into nurse practice	Follows evidence-based medication administration delivery system
Follows established standards of patient care	Maintains sterile technique for invasive procedures
Knowledgeable care delivery	Holds specialty nursing certification
Actively participates in care evaluation processes	Performs root cause analysis to determine medication error rate with nurses working overtime
Participates in quality enhancement data collection	Completes quality improvement audits for documentation of timely electrocardiogram interpretations

interest of the patient while simultaneously acknowledging and respecting the important role of the family. Critical care nurses round with physicians, attend interdisciplinary patient care conferences, and interpret health information in a way that can be understood by patients and their families.[22] **Box 3** lists significant advocacy roles for the critical care nurse.

Model of Professional Nursing Regulation

Nurses must deliver safe and effective complex care. The public also has this expectation. The identified psychosocial outcomes supported by critical care nurses of holistic care, coping, community reintegration, knowledge, quality care (delivery), and advocacy are hallmarks for the Model of Professional Regulation.[23] Critical care nurses maintain their scope of practice by following the steps within this model.

Nursing is a highly regulated professional discipline and state boards of nursing assure the public that nurses are competent to practice. RNs must hold valid licensure through state and/or territorial regulatory bodies. Regulation is accomplished through rules and regulations for state licensure standards for clinical nursing practice, an established code of ethics, nursing specialty certification, agency policies, protocols and procedures, and the nurse's self-determination. Nurses are independently responsible for assuring their self-determination. Self-determination mandates that the nurse be accountable in maintaining autonomy within their scope of practice. This is accomplished through maintaining professional licensure and specialty certification, securing high knowledge levels through conference attendance, participating in workshops, earning continuing education units, placing current evidence into nurse practice, and inviting peer review.[23]

The Model of Professional Regulation builds in complexity from the lowest level depicting the professional standards of practice, scope of nursing practice, the code of ethics and specialty certification to the top level of the model, self-determination, in which the nurse must apply all levels of the pyramid. Self-determination supports that the nurse who applies earlier steps in the model is an autonomous, independent decision-maker.[23] This means that the nurse can follow or not follow a physician's order. Nurses, using their clinical judgment, can elect not to follow a physician's order is they believe that it would create an unsafe circumstance and negatively impact quality care delivery.

The Model of Professional Regulation is guided by 3 major concepts: quality, safety, and evidence. ICU nurses must maintain vigilance when using advanced technologies,

---

Box 3
Advocacy roles for nurses practicing in intensive care units

- Be a voice for patients who cannot speak
- Act as an advocate or liaison between the patient, family, provider, and health care team, and intercede when necessary
- Promote quality care through upholding established standards of care
- Uphold patient decisions
- Provide information or education to the patient and/or their family so that informed decisions can be made
- Respect patient privacy for medical information and personal care provision
- Respect the patients cultural values and beliefs

communicating care treatments, and managing challenges unique to critically ill patients at any age who present with multiple comorbidities and may be facing end-of-life decisions.[23]

SUMMARY

Critical care nurses have a pivotal role in provision of psychosocial care that improves and supports psychosocial outcomes. ICU environments contribute to stressors that challenge critical care nurses to provide personalized care that promotes privacy in often noisy and impersonal settings. Psychosocial care by nursing staff is reinforced by the ANA Code of Ethics, which promulgates treating patients and their families with dignity, respect, and a holistic overall approach to care delivery. Educating the patient, explaining procedures, and practicing sound communication skills represents higher levels of psychosocial care. Time invested in staff development sessions for ICU nursing personnel for therapeutic use of psychosocial care approaches will positively improve psychosocial outcomes. These management strategies can significantly increase patient and family well-being in adjusting to discharge into the home, community, or long-term care facility.[4,8,9,16,17] Consequently, hospital leaders should take stock and incorporate psychosocial care management strategies into their critical care units that improve psychosocial outcomes.

REFERENCES

1. Breenan M. Gallup Poll Web site. Nurses again outpace other professions for honesty, ethics. Available at: https://news.gallup.com/poll/245597/nurses-again-outpace-professions-honesty-ethics.aspx. Accessed February 10, 2019.
2. Breenan M. Gallup Poll Web site. Nurses keep healthy lead on most honest, ethical profession. Available at: https://nurse.org/articles/gallup-ethical-standards-poll-nurses-rank-highest/. Accessed February 10, 2019.
3. American Association of Critical Care Nurses. AACN scope and standards for acute and critical care nursing practice. Aliso Viejo (CA): American Association of Critical Care Nurses; 2015.
4. Hamstra B. 4 major differences between ICU and emergency nurses. Available at: https://nurse.org/articles/differences-between-icu-er-nurses/. Accessed February 7, 2019.
5. Urden LD, Stacy KM, Lough ME. Priorities in critical care nursing. Priorities in critical care nursing. 8th edition. St Louis (MO): Elsevier; 2019.
6. Chivukula U, Hariharan M, Suvashisa R, et al. Role of psychosocial care on ICU trauma. Indian J Psychol Med 2014;36(3):312–6.
7. American Nurses Association. Code of ethics for with interpretative statements. Silver Springs (MD): Nursesbooks.org; 2015.
8. Heyland DK, Rocker GM, Dodek PM, et al. Family satisfaction with care in the intensive care unit: results of a multiple center study. Crit Care Med 2002;30(7): 1413–8.
9. Leske J. Needs of family members after critical illness: prescriptions for interventions. Crit Care Nurs Clin North Am 1993;4(4):587–96.
10. Chaing VL, Chien WT, Wong HT, et al. A Brief Cognitive-Behavioral Psycho-Education (B-CBE) program for managing stress and anxiety of main family caregivers of patients in intensive care unit. Int J Environ Res Public Health 2016; 13(962):1–13.

11. Parker AM, Sricharoenchai T, Needham DM. Early rehabilitation in the intensive care unit: preventing impairment of physical and mental health. Curr Phys Med Rehabil Rep 2013;1(4):307–14.
12. Garrouste-Orgeas M, Coquet I, Perier A, et al. Impact of an intensive care unit diary on psychological distress in the patients and relatives. Crit Care Med 2012; 40:2033–40.
13. Nydahl P. ICU-diary. Web site. 2012. Available at: http://www.icu-diary.org. Accessed February 25, 2019.
14. Chivukula U, Hariharan M, Rana S, et al. Enhancing hospital well-being and minimizing intensive care unit trauma: cushioning effects of psychosocial care. Indian J Crit Care Med 2017;21(10):640–5.
15. Kotfits K, Marra A, Ely EW. ICU delirium: a diagnostic and therapeutic challenge in the intensive care unit. Anaesthesiol Intensive Ther 2018;50(2):128–40.
16. Gerber L. Understanding the nurse's role as a patient advocate. Nursing 2018; 48(4):55–8.
17. Walker DK, Barton-Burke M, Saria MG, et al. Everyday advocates: nursing advocacy is a full-time job. Am J Nurs 2015;115(8):66–70.
18. Choii PP. Patient advocacy: the role of the nurse. Nurs Stand 2015;29(41):52–8.
19. Zolnierek C. Speak to be heard: effective nurse advocacy. Am Nurse Today 2012; 7:10.
20. Nursing: scope and standards of practice. 2nd edition. Silver Spring (MD): American Nurses Association; 2010.
21. Davoodvand S, Abbaszaheh A, Ahmadi F. Patient Advocacy from the clinical nurses' viewpoint: a qualitative study. J Med Ethics Hist Med 2016;9:5.
22. Fahlberg B, Dickmann C. Promoting family advocacy. Nursing 2015;45(8):14–5.
23. Styles MM, Schumann MJ, Bickford C, et al. Specialization and credentialing in nursing revisited: understanding the issues, advancing the profession. Silver Spring (MD): American Nurses Association; 2008.

Psychological Issues of Patient Transition from Intensive Care to Palliative Care

Dorothy Wholihan, DNP, AGPCNP-BC, GNP-BC, ACHPN, FPCN

KEYWORDS

- Palliative care • End-of-life transitions • Goals of care • Psychological issues

KEY POINTS

- Transitions of goals of care in the intensive care unit (ICU) from life-prolonging aggressive treatment to comfort-oriented care can be fraught with psychological stress.
- As intimate bedside caregivers, nurses are well suited to facilitate decisions to transition care.
- Effective empathic communication is integral to clarifying values and facilitating smooth transitions of care.
- Early integration of specialty palliative care in the ICU is beneficial to patients, families, and staff.

FOCUS OF CARE IN THE INTENSIVE CARE UNIT

Intensive care units (ICUs) came into existence in the 1950s, along with the rapid development of complex medical therapies and technologies aimed at saving the most critically ill patients in an arena where expertise and technology could be concentrated.[1] The primary goals of aggressive ICU care are patient resuscitation and the stabilizing and recovery of patients after a serious acute event, yet many patients do die in the ICU.[2] Analysis of Medicare data has shown that there is a significant increase in the use of intensive care before death, with 29% of patients spending time in an ICU in the month before their death.[3]

This life-saving mission has not changed, yet the changing demographics of the population have led to more elderly and frail chronically ill patients surviving for long periods with the assistance of intensive care. These chronically critically ill patients experience a complex syndrome of physiologic alterations, consume significant resources, and present significant challenges to clinicians. Their number is expected to increase more than 5.5% each year, as the population ages.[4] Despite intensive

Disclosure: The author has nothing to disclose.
NYU Meyers College of Nursing, 433 First Avenue, New York, NY 10010, USA
E-mail address: dw57@nyu.edu

technological life-prolonging treatment, progression of their underlying conditions continues and death is an inevitable outcome.

Patients and families frequently experience psychological trauma from extended hospitalizations in intensive care settings, including anxiety, depression, and posttraumatic stress disorder (PTSD).[5,6] There also are significant psychological consequences when families and patients must face the decision to change the focus of care away from aggressive life-prolonging treatment toward comfort-oriented care, and nurses can play an integral role in easing this transition.[7]

TRANSITIONS TO END-OF-LIFE CARE IN THE INTENSIVE CARE UNIT

Transitioning away from life-prolonging care is an uncomfortable experience for patients, families, and care providers. The first step for the health care team is to acknowledge the reality of the clinical situation: that aggressive intensive treatment will not have a positive impact on patient outcomes and may, in fact, be increasing suffering. This realization that life-prolonging goals will not be met may lead to feelings of failure on the part of the medical team. Even if a patient's condition is a result of overwhelming pathology, it is common, especially for medical providers, to feel inadequate when patients look to them for life-saving answers that they cannot provide. Frustration, defensiveness, and anxiety may subsequently play into the picture. A strong team can help recognize these feelings and support one another during these uncomfortable times. Personal reflection and collaborative support are essential to maintain the emotional health of caregivers facing difficult care transitions and painful discussions with patient or family. Successful support of patients and families requires support for each other.

THE NURSE AS FACILITATOR IN THE TRANSITION

Nurses spend the most time of any health professional in direct contact with patients and families; they are involved with intimate care and are present at the most vulnerable moments. As such, critical care nurses at the bedside are well placed to facilitate discussions of patient and family values in relation to treatment decisions.

They frequently prompt family discussions and referrals to palliative care.[7] Critical care nurses also frequently act as mediators among patients and families and the myriad levels of interprofessional medical staff involved in the complex care of these severely ill patients. Qualitative nursing literature describes numerous communication strategies utilized by experienced nurses when addressing withdrawal of aggressive treatment; Peden-McAlpine and colleagues[8] analyzed 7 descriptive studies of communication strategies and categorized them into 4 elements: general communication and relationship building, recognizing the need to transition to palliative care, facilitating palliative care, and providing dignified care to death. Broom and colleagues[7] interviewed 20 nurses to explore the complex roles of nurses in facilitating transitions to palliative care. They report that nurses view themselves as ideally placed to advocate for patients to specialists who are more focused on clinical status and life-prolonging treatment as opposed to psychosocial and supportive care. According to these researchers, nursing expertise is centered on the big picture, the backstage of the patient experience: "what is really going on" and "how they are really coping" to ascertain if specialty palliative care referrals might be needed.[7]

In the transition away from aggressive therapy, nurses at the bedside often are the first ones to recognize that patients are approaching death.[9] They then frequently facilitate family recognition of declining status, and, in an advocacy role, they then move on to help navigate communication among patient, family, and medical staff.[10]

Obviously, time from ICU entrance to acceptance of pending death (with appropriate withdrawal of treatment) varies with the clinical situation. In cases of a severe trauma with overwhelming injury, family may have only hours until their loved one dies, whereas in cases of multiple medical chronic comorbidities, patients may linger for weeks or even months. It is imperative that nurses remain sensitive to the timing of such transitions and the emotional reactions and needs of patients and families.[2] Transitions in ICU are also frequently challenging because clear prognostication and high risk for death prediction is not always possible.[11] Again, nurses can facilitate discussion of underlying values and goals to clarify what is most important to patients and families in any given situation.

Adding to the complexity concerning discussion of care transition is the emotional impact on the involved health care providers. Communication experts Back and colleagues[12(p108)] write:

> No matter how important or appropriate it is to shift the goals of care from extending life to providing comfort, the fact remains the talking about transitions means that the medicine [or technology] is not working, and this invokes disappointment, loss and sadness. These conversations force patients and families to confront the failure of medical treatments, their own failures, and existential and spiritual crises. All these dimensions make talking about transitions very complex and ridden with emotion.

At times, nurses must intercede on behalf of patients with medical colleagues who are reluctant to accept that it may be time for withdrawal of aggressive care. In these instances, nurses must carefully negotiate the environment of medical dominance in the hospital system. They must take up the role of intimate mediator, which can carry an interprofessional cost and cause significant stress within the ICU system.[7]

COMMUNICATION STRATEGIES

Unfortunately, complex communication skills have not often been adequately taught to those preparing for the health professions, and many clinicians feel ill prepared for serious discussions about transitions away from aggressive care.[13]

Discussing goals of care is much more than the completion of an advance directive or a decision regarding cardiopulmonary resuscitation. This type of care planning is a process, not a document. As such, it involves an exploration of patient and family values and getting to know patients and families on a deeper level. A palliative care focus changes the conversation from "What's the matter with you?" to "What matters to you?" Without an underlying understanding of the patient and family, simple recommendation of a change in goals can be unsuccessful. Exploration of values is integral to the process.[12]

Several models exist to assist clinicians to frame these difficult conversations about transitions away from aggressive care to comfort-oriented care. These include the SPIKES model for breaking bad news,[13] NURSE statements to facilitate the response to strong emotion,[12] and the REMAP model for discussion of changing goals of care.[14] These mnemonic models are detailed in **Table 1**.

Many nurses are afraid to discuss care transitions and end-of-life care for fear that they will increase suffering or unleash emotions in patients or families that they are ill equipped to handle. Fear, sadness, anger, and frustration are all common responses to serious news. The role of the clinician in addressing these emotions is to provide a safe space of nonjudgment and support by maintaining a trusting therapeutic partnership and to not worsen the experience by minimizing the emotion.[15] Rather, validation,

Table 1 Useful communication tools		
Model		**Description and/or Example**
SPIKES	S: setting	Create privacy, be prepared.
Model for breaking	P: perception	"What is your understanding....?"
bad news	I: invitation	"How would you like information to be delivered?"
	K: knowledge	Impart information gently; avoid jargon, use warning shot.
	E: emotion	Respond to strong emotion.
	S: summary	Summarize; teach-back, plan.
REMAP	R: reframe	Discuss need to re-evaluate plan.
Model for discussing	E: emotion	Expect emotion; use reflective statements.
goals of care	M: map	Step back and explore values.
	A: align	Summarize values and goals.
	P: plan	Propose a plan reflecting values.
NURSE	N: naming	"It sounds like..."
Statements to respond	U: understanding	"What I understand you to be saying..."
to strong emotion	R: respecting	"I am impressed by..."
	S: supporting	"We are here for you..."
	E: Exploring	"Can you tell me more...?"

Data from Refs.[12–14]

understanding, exploration, and support are all therapeutic responses. Naming the emotion, "This situation is really upsetting," validates the patient/family experience and expresses empathy. Silence also is a powerful tool. In a study of ICU family meetings, when empathic statements were followed by a pause, rather than additional information, family members were 18-fold more likely to share concerns, hopes, or values.[16] The acronym NURSE is an exceptional tool to assist nurses and other clinicians in responding to strong emotions expected when patients face the end of their lives.

COMMUNICATION TRAINING

Communication skills, like any other clinical practice, can be taught and improved with practice. Several training programs have been established across the country. An example is the VitalTalk program, which presents many useful tools.[17] The End-of-Life Nursing Education Consortium (ELNEC) emphasizes communication training in all its programs and has a course specifically geared toward palliative care in the ICU named ELNEC Critical Care.[18]

ELNEC also has developed a national train-the-trainer program specifically designed to disseminate communication training and is useful in detailing many effective communication strategies.[19] All of these resources also include specific strategies for dealing with formal family meetings. Online resources for communication training are listed in **Box 1**.

FAMILY MEETINGS

Family meetings can be the most useful tool in communicating status, prognosis, and compassion to families, but the therapeutic value of the family meeting can be greatly enhanced if these interactions can focus on listening to family perspectives values rather than merely imparting information. Laurette and colleagues[20] tested an intervention they titled, the VALUE family meeting. This large randomized control trial, which included 22 ICUs throughout France, tested a structured family meeting tool as well as a bereavement brochure. The VALUE family meeting structure emphasized family members rather than providers speaking for most of the time. Empathic listening and support were emphasized. The framework is presented in **Box 2**.

Follow-up phone interviews found that longer family meetings (median 30 min vs 20 min) and meetings in which the majority of time was spent listening to families (median 14 vs 5 min) resulted in families experiencing less guilt and able to withdraw aggressive therapies, like pressors and mechanical ventilation. Furthermore, families in the VALUE intervention meetings reported less anxiety, depression, and PTSD symptoms.

It is widely recognized that family meetings should be held early after ICU admission to ascertain patient and family knowledge of patient condition as well as goals and preferences.[21] Many recommend that meetings be held within 5 days, at the least.[2] Although daily updates are always appropriate, a formal meeting to elucidate goals should be held early and repeated as the patient condition changes.

COMPLEX TRANSITIONAL SITUATIONS
Hope for a Miracle

Family members may hold out what is perceived as unrealistic hope and resist all attempts to transition patients away from aggressive life-prolonging care. The hope for a miracle may emanate from feelings of hopelessness and desperation as well as a deep religious faith; it can become the ultimate treatment options when all other therapy fails.[22] It is recommended to not fight or confront a family's expressions of hopefulness. Using "wish" statements can be useful in this situation: "I wish I could promise that things would get better. I hope he gets better soon too."[2(p747)] Cooper and colleagues[23] propose a 4-step response to challenging conversations about miracles that they name, the AMEN protocol, which involves validating the patient/family belief system, meeting them where they are, educating them about medical issues, and reassuring them about nonabandonment.

The AMEN protocol is presented in **Box 3**.

The premise of advance care planning is to hope for the best but prepare for the worst.[24] Hopes can be reframed; they change as illness progresses. Hope for a full recovery may change to hope for other things: opportunities to see family milestones, such as birthdays or weddings, and the ability to reconnect with family, to return home, or to finish unresolved personal issues.[25]

Pediatric Care

Perhaps the most difficult population for care planning discussion is within the pediatric arena. Care providers often worry about overwhelming parents with these

---

Box 1
Resources for communication skills training

VitalTalk: https://www.vitaltalk.org/

ELNEC: https://www.aacnnursing.org/ELNEC

International Association for Communication in Healthcare: http://www.each.eu/teaching/resources/

Stanford School of Medicine http://palliative.stanford.edu/communication-breaking-bad-news/

American Association of Critical-Care Nurses webinar series: https://www.aacn.org/education/webinar-series

---

Box 2
VALUE family meeting objectives

- Value and appreciate what family said.
- Acknowledge family emotions.
- Listen.
- Understand the patient as person.
- Elicit questions from family members.

Data from Laurette, A, Darmon, M, Megarbane, B, et al. A communication strategy and brochure for relatives of patients dying in the ICU. New Engl J Med. 2007;356(5):469–78.

---

emotion-laden discussions. Lotz and colleagues[26] conducted a qualitative review of family members whose child had died of a serious illness. The researchers found that family did report great difficulty discussing goals and care planning, but parents viewed it as important and recommended a sensitive, gradual, individualized patient-centered and family-centered approach in which hope and quality of life remained key issues.

Surrogate Decision Makers

Frequently, in critical care settings, patients are severely ill or lack decision-making capacity and cannot participate in determining their own goals or plans of care. In these instances, health care providers must rely on family members or proxy surrogates. These situations may present complicated decision making, especially if families are conflicted or have been out of touch with the patient, a phenomenon actually named, the Daughter from California Syndrome.[27] Ideally, an advance directive may be in place to guide decisions, or at the least, a proxy has been established who has communicated with the patient. Unfortunately, the rate of completion for advance directives remains low.[2,28] So, frequently, clinicians must rely on surrogates to make decisions based on substituted judgment, yet surrogates do not always have a clear understanding of a patient's wishes. In these instances, referral to palliative care specialists often can help clarify these wishes and often help resolve any conflict that may arise.[29]

ROLE OF A PALLIATIVE CARE CONSULTATION

Given the life-saving orientation of intensive care, palliative care may seem inconsistent with the critical care environment. Seriously acutely ill patients, however, have

---

Box 3
The AMEN response to hope in miracles

A: Affirm the patient/family belief system.

M: Meet the patient/family where they are.

E: Educate the patient/family regarding medical status and facts.

N: *"No matter what…"*; assure nonabandonment.

Data from Cooper, RS, Ferguson, A. Bodurtha, JN, Smith, TJ. AMEN in challenging conversations: Bridging the gaps between faith, hope and medicine. J Oncol Pract. 2014;10(4)e191–95.

---

myriad palliative needs. According to the 2018 guidelines developed by the National Consensus Project, palliative care focuses on expert pain and symptom management, assessment, and support of caregiver needs and coordination of care. It is a person-centered and family-centered approach, attending to the physical, psychological, practical, and spiritual consequences of any serious illness.[30] The basic principles of palliative care are outlined in **Box 4**.

All providers are encouraged to obtain the core skills needed to incorporate basic palliative care into their practice. This primary palliative care can be provided by any clinician or interdisciplinary provider.[31] Patients and families with complex needs or the presence of conflicting goals of care may benefit from the help of specialty palliative care, provided by a skilled, interdisciplinary team of national board-certified palliative experts.

Knowing when and how to consult palliative care specialists can be a complicated issue. Although specialty palliative care has been proved to improve quality of life and reduce cost,[32] the actual consultation of the palliative care team can be challenging for intensivists managing the care of such patients. Introducing palliative care results in patient and family resistance to the transition, bringing to light the clinical uncertainty of prognostication and the question of medical futility, and general resistance on the part of all, as a result of everyone's need to retain hope.[33] Some patients and families gain relief, however, when life-prolonging treatment ceases and care focused on comfort and quality of life begins.[34] Broom and colleagues,[33] in their descriptive study of communication by primary physicians introducing palliative care, report that such conversations must entail a multidimensional consideration of the whole patient/family, from biographic, social, and cultural perspectives. Early integration of palliative care in the advanced cancer population has shown substantial impact on quality of life and quality of end-of-life care.[35] It can be extrapolated that earlier integration in the ICU will also provide the ongoing support needed to ease end-of-life transitions.

SUPPORTING INTENSIVE CARE CLINICIANS

There is a plethora of studies demonstrating the stress and caregiver fatigue that emanates from the tension resulting from perceived overly burdensome cure-oriented care in the ICU.[2] If left out of care discussions and family meetings, the bedside nurse can be at serious high risk for moral distress. Strategies, such as debriefing and sharing narratives, can create supportive bonds among all disciplines. Recognizing patients as individuals can help reinforce the underlying compassion and personhood

---

Box 4
Characteristics of palliative care

1. Appropriate at any stage of serious illness, regardless of setting, diagnosis, prognosis, or age

2. Beneficial when provided along with curative life-prolonging treatment

3. Offered in all are settings and health care systems

4. Interdisciplinary care to attend to holistic needs of patients and families

5. Focusing on and working toward goals and preferences most important to patient and family

Data from National Consensus Project for Quality Palliative Care. clinical practice guidelines for quality palliative care. 4th ed.. Richmond, VA: National Coalition for Hospice and Palliative Care. 2018. Available at: https://www.nationalcoalitionhpc.org/ncp Accessed Feb 27, 2019.

of providers. Providence Health & Services in Washington State developed a practice known as The Pause. A poignant video illustrates the inclusion of this moment of silence and reflection on clinician efforts in a critical situation (https://www.youtube.com/watch?v=_HVXM2YhZ2A). This practice has been integrated in some intensive care settings. Inclusion of all significant staff, especially nurses involved in direct care, in family meetings and decision-making discussions can help minimize distress and burnout in these ICU caregivers by allowing the entire picture of medicine-family interactions and allowing contributions to care discussions.

End-of-life care in the ICU is fraught with complicated psychological responses by patients, families, and staff. Empathic and mindful communication, inclusion of all integral staff in decision-making meetings, and multidimensional support of patients and families can ease the transition away from aggressive life-prolonging to comfort-oriented care.

REFERENCES

1. Wiencek C. Palliative care in the intensive care unit setting. In: Dahlin C, Coyne PJ, Ferrell BR, editors. Advanced practice palliative nursing. New York: Oxford University Press; 2016. p. 65–73.
2. McAdam J, Puntillo K. The intensive care unit. In: Ferrell BR, Coyle N, Paice JA, editors. Oxford textbook of palliative nursing. 4th edition. New York: Oxford University Press; 2015. p. 740–60.
3. Miesfeldt S, Murray K, Lucas L, et al. Change in end-of-life care for Medicare beneficiaries: site of death, place of care, and health care transitions in 2000, 2005, and 2009. JAMA 2012;309(5):470–7.
4. Nelson JE, Cox CE, Hope A, et al. Chronic critical illness: prevalence, profile, and pathophsyiology. AACN Adv Crit Care 2010;21(10):44–61.
5. McAdam JL, Fontaine DK, While DB, et al. Psychological symptoms of family of high-risk intensive care unit patients. Am J Crit Care 2012;21(6):386–94.
6. Fumis RRL, Ranzini OT, Martins PS, et al. Emotional disorders in pairs of patients and their family member during and after ICU stay. PLoS One 2015;10(1): e0115332. Available at: https://journals.plos.org/plosone/article/file?id=10.1371/journal.pone.0115332&type=printable. Accessed March 5, 2019.
7. Broom A, Kirby E, Good P, et al. Negotiating futility, managing emotions: nursing the transition to palliative care. Qual Health Res 2015;25(3):299–309.
8. Peden-McAlpine C, Liaschenko J, Traudt T. Constructing the story: how nurses work with families regarding withdrawal of aggressive treatment in ICU- A narrative study. Int J Nurs Stud 2015;52:1146–56.
9. Bach V, Ploeg J, Black M. Nursing roles in end-of-life decision-making in critical care settings. West J Nurs Res 2009;31(4):496–512.
10. Gutierrez KM. Prognostic communication of critical care nurses and physicians at end of life. Dimens Crit Care Nurs 2012;31(3):170–82.
11. Fisher M, Ridley S. Uncertainty in end-of-life care and shared decision making. Crit Care Resusc 2012;14(1):81–7.
12. Back A, Arnold R, Tulsky J. Mastering communication with seriously ill patients: balancing honesty with empathy and hope. New York: Cambridge University Press; 2010.
13. Baile WF, Buckman R, Lenzi R, et al. SPIKES – a six-step protocol for delivering bad news: application to the patient with cancer. Oncologist 2012;5:302–11.
14. Childers JW, Back AL, Tulsky JA, et al. REMAP: a framework for goals of care conversations. J Oncol Pract 2017;13(10):e844–50.

15. Weissman DE, Quill TE, Arnold RM. Fast facts and concepts # 24: responding to emotion in family meetings. 2015. Available at: http://www.mypcnow.org/blank-k4ibb. Accessed March 1, 2019.

16. October TW, Dizon ZB, Arnold RM, et al. Characteristics of physician empathetic statements during pediatric intensive care conferences with family members: a qualitative study. JAMA Netw Open 2018;1(3):1–11.

17. Vital Talk. Responding to emotion: articulating empathy using NURSE statements. Available at: http://vitaltalk.org/guides/responding-to-emotion-respecting/. Accessed March 3, 2019.

18. Grant M, Wiencek C, Virani R, et al. End-of-life care education in acute and critical care: the California ELNEC project. AACN Adv Crit Care 2013;24(2):121–9.

19. Bulller H, Virani R, Malloy P, et al. End-of-life nursing and education consortium communication curriculum. J Hosp Palliat Nurs 2019;21(2):e5–12.

20. Laurette A, Darmon M, Megarbane B, et al. A communication strategy and brochure for relatives of patients dying in the ICU. N Engl J Med 2007;356: 469–78.

21. Nelson JE, Walker AS, Luhrs CA, et al. Family meetings made simpler: a toolkit for the intensive care unit. J Crit Care 2009;24(40):626.e7-14.

22. Cooper RS, Knight L, Ferguson A. Trust, hope and miracles. In: Wittenberg E, Ferrell BR, Goldsmith J, et al, editors. Textbook of palliative care communication. New York: Oxford University Press; 2016. p. 255–62.

23. Cooper RS, Ferguson A, Bodurtha JN, et al. AMEN in challenging conversations: bridging the gaps between faith, hope and medicine. J Oncol Pract 2014;10(4): e191–5.

24. Thurston A, Arnold R. Insight and information are key to implementing palliative care. Today's Geriatric Med 2015;8(4):16.

25. Boreale K. Communication. In: Coyne PJ, Bobb B, Plakovic K, editors. Conversations in palliative care. 2nd edition. Pittsburgh (PA): Hospice and Palliative Nurses Association; 2017. p. 33–46.

26. Lotz JD, Daxer M, Jox RJ, et al. "Hope for the best, prepare for the worst": a qualitative interview study on parents' needs and fears in pediatric advance care planning. Palliat Med 2017;3(8):764–71.

27. Unger T. The daughter from California syndrome. Palliat Med 2010;13(12):1405.

28. Halpern NA, Pastores SM, Chou JF, et al. Advance directives in an oncologic intensive care unit: a contemporary analysis of their frequency, type and impact. J Palliat Med 2011;14(4):483–9.

29. Thurston A, Fettig L, Arnold R. Team communication in the acute care setting. In: Wittenberg E, Ferrell BR, Goldsmith J, et al, editors. Textbook of palliative care communication. New York: Oxford University Press; 2016. p. 321–9.

30. NCP (national Consensus Project for quality palliative care). Clinical practice guidelines for quality palliative care. 4th edition. Richmond (VA): National Coalition for Hospice and Palliative Care; 2018. Available at: https://www.nationalcoalitionhpc.org/ncp. Accessed Feb 27, 2019.

31. IOM (Institute of Medicine). Dying in America: improving quality and honoring preferences near the end of life. Washington, DC: The National Academies Press; 2015. Available at: https://www.nap.edu/catalog/18748/dying-in-america-improving-quality-and-honoring-individual-preferences-near. Accessed March 1, 2019.

32. Kyeremanteng K, Gagnin L, Thavorn K, et al. The impact of palliative care consultation in the ICU on length of stay: a systematic review and cost evaluation. J Intensive Care Med 2018;33(6):346–53.

33. Broom A, Kirby E, Good P, et al. The trouble of telling: managing communication about the end of life. Qual Health Res 2014;24(2):151–62.
34. Campbell T, Carey E, Jackson V, et al. Discussing prognosis: balancing hope and realism. Cancer J 2010;16:461–6.
35. Temel JS, Greer JA, Muzikansky A, et al. Early palliative care for patients with metastatic non-small cell lung cancer. N Engl J Med 2010;363:733–42.

UNITED STATES POSTAL SERVICE® Statement of Ownership, Management, and Circulation (All Periodicals Publications Except Requester Publications)

1. Publication Title	2. Publication Number	3. Filing Date
CRITICAL CARE NURSING CLINICS OF NORTH AMERICA	006 — 273	9/18/19

4. Issue Frequency	5. Number of Issues Published Annually	6. Annual Subscription Price
MAR, JUN SEP, DEC	4	$160.00

7. Complete Mailing Address of Known Office of Publication (Not printer) (Street, city, county, state, and ZIP+4®)

ELSEVIER INC.
230 Park Avenue, Suite 800
New York, NY 10169

Contact Person
STEPHEN R. BUSHING

Telephone (Include area code)
215-239-3688

8. Complete Mailing Address of Headquarters or General Business Office of Publisher (Not printer)

ELSEVIER INC.
230 Park Avenue, Suite 800
New York, NY 10169

9. Full Names and Complete Mailing Addresses of Publisher, Editor, and Managing Editor (Do not leave blank)

Publisher (Name and complete mailing address)

TAYLOR BALL, ELSEVIER INC.
1600 JOHN F KENNEDY BLVD. SUITE 1800
PHILADELPHIA, PA 19103-2899

Editor (Name and complete mailing address)

KERRY HOLLAND, ELSEVIER INC.
1600 JOHN F KENNEDY BLVD. SUITE 1800
PHILADELPHIA, PA 19103-2899

Managing Editor (Name and complete mailing address)

PATRICK MANLEY, ELSEVIER INC.
1600 JOHN F KENNEDY BLVD. SUITE 1800
PHILADELPHIA, PA 19103-2899

10. Owner (Do not leave blank. If the publication is owned by a corporation, give the name and address of the corporation immediately followed by the names and addresses of all stockholders owning or holding 1 percent or more of the total amount of stock. If not owned by a corporation, give the names and addresses of the individual owners. If owned by a partnership or other unincorporated firm, give its name and address as well as those of each individual owner. If the publication is published by a nonprofit organization, give its name and address.)

Full Name	Complete Mailing Address
WHOLLY OWNED SUBSIDIARY OF REED/ELSEVIER, US HOLDINGS	1600 JOHN F KENNEDY BLVD. SUITE 1800 PHILADELPHIA, PA 19103-2899

11. Known Bondholders, Mortgagees, and Other Security Holders Owning or Holding 1 Percent or More of Total Amount of Bonds, Mortgages, or Other Securities. If none, check box ▶ ☐ None

Full Name	Complete Mailing Address
N/A	

12. Tax Status (For completion by nonprofit organizations authorized to mail at nonprofit rates) (Check one)
The purpose, function, and nonprofit status of this organization and the exempt status for federal income tax purposes:
☒ Has Not Changed During Preceding 12 Months
☐ Has Changed During Preceding 12 Months (Publisher must submit explanation of change with this statement)

PS Form **3526**, July 2014 [Page 1 of 4 (see instructions page 4)] PSN 7530-01-000-9931 PRIVACY NOTICE: See our privacy policy on www.usps.com.

13. Publication Title	14. Issue Date for Circulation Data Below
CRITICAL CARE NURSING CLINICS OF NORTH AMERICA	JUNE 2019

15. Extent and Nature of Circulation		Average No. Copies Each Issue During Preceding 12 Months	No. Copies of Single Issue Published Nearest to Filing Date
a. Total Number of Copies (Net press run)		147	143
b. Paid Circulation (By Mail and Outside the Mail)	(1) Mailed Outside-County Paid Subscriptions Stated on PS Form 3541 (Include paid distribution above nominal rate, advertiser's proof copies, and exchange copies)	73	78
	(2) Mailed In-County Paid Subscriptions Stated on PS Form 3541 (Include paid distribution above nominal rate, advertiser's proof copies, and exchange copies)	0	0
	(3) Paid Distribution Outside the Mails Including Sales Through Dealers and Carriers, Street Vendors, Counter Sales, and Other Paid Distribution Outside USPS®	26	29
	(4) Paid Distribution by Other Classes of Mail Through the USPS (e.g. First-Class Mail®)	0	0
c. Total Paid Distribution (Sum of 15b (1), (2), (3), and (4))		99	107
d. Free or Nominal Rate Distribution (By Mail and Outside the Mail)	(1) Free or Nominal Rate Outside-County Copies Included on PS Form 3541	37	21
	(2) Free or Nominal Rate In-County Copies Included on PS Form 3541	0	0
	(3) Free or Nominal Rate Copies Mailed at Other Classes Through the USPS (e.g. First-Class Mail)	0	0
	(4) Free or Nominal Rate Distribution Outside the Mail (Carriers or other means)	0	0
e. Total Free or Nominal Rate Distribution (Sum of 15d (1), (2), (3) and (4))		37	21
f. Total Distribution (Sum of 15c and 15e)		136	128
g. Copies not Distributed (See Instructions to Publishers #4 (page 83))		11	15
h. Total (Sum of 15f and g)		147	143
i. Percent Paid (15c divided by 15f times 100)		72.79%	83.6%

* If you are claiming electronic copies, go to line 16 on page 3. If you are not claiming electronic copies, skip to line 17 on page 3.

PS Form **3526**, July 2014 (Page 2 of 4)

16. Electronic Copy Circulation	Average No. Copies Each Issue During Preceding 12 Months	No. Copies of Single Issue Published Nearest to Filing Date
a. Paid Electronic Copies ▶		
b. Total Paid Print Copies (Line 15c) + Paid Electronic Copies (Line 16a) ▶		
c. Total Print Distribution (Line 15f) + Paid Electronic Copies (Line 16a) ▶		
d. Percent Paid (Both Print & Electronic Copies) (16b divided by 16c × 100) ▶		

☒ I certify that 50% of all my distributed copies (electronic and print) are paid above a nominal price.

17. Publication of Statement of Ownership
☒ If the publication is a general publication, publication of this statement is required. Will be printed ☐ Publication not required.
in the DECEMBER 2019 issue of this publication.

18. Signature and Title of Editor, Publisher, Business Manager, or Owner

STEPHEN R. BUSHING, INVENTORY DISTRIBUTION CONTROL MANAGER

Stephen R. Bushing

Date 9/18/19

I certify that all information furnished on this form is true and complete. I understand that anyone who furnishes false or misleading information on this form or who omits material or information requested on the form may be subject to criminal sanctions (including fines and imprisonment) and/or civil sanctions (including civil penalties).

PS Form **3526**, July 2014 (Page 3 of 4) PRIVACY NOTICE: See our privacy policy on www.usps.com.

Moving?

Make sure your subscription moves with you!

To notify us of your new address, find your **Clinics Account Number** (located on your mailing label above your name), and contact customer service at:

Email: journalscustomerservice-usa@elsevier.com

800-654-2452 (subscribers in the U.S. & Canada)
314-447-8871 (subscribers outside of the U.S. & Canada)

Fax number: 314-447-8029

Elsevier Health Sciences Division
Subscription Customer Service
3251 Riverport Lane
Maryland Heights, MO 63043

*To ensure uninterrupted delivery of your subscription, please notify us at least 4 weeks in advance of move.

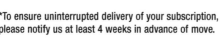

Printed and bound by CPI Group (UK) Ltd, Croydon, CR0 4YY

03/10/2024

01040484-0013